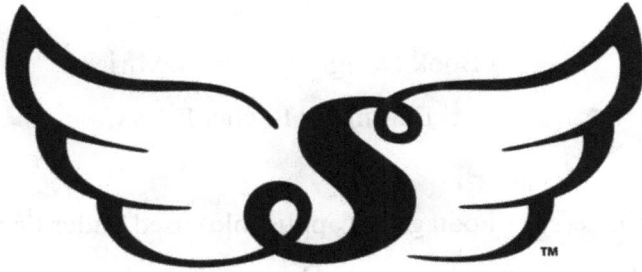

SOULFIT

4th Edition – 2025

Dedication

I dedicate this book to our father and the king of the universe. Second, my amazing wife, who has sacrificed herself beyond measure. Her reward is priceless. I thank my parents, Aryeh Leon and Zahava, for their love and discipline in my upbringing throughout childhood. My Rabbis, teachers, coaches, friends, family, and mentors have educated me and taken the time to teach me the Torah and its hidden meanings and teachings. They also pulled me up when I was down and listened to me when I needed them, too, all my loyal friends and family, believing in the big picture. Finally dedicated to you, the truth-seeking passionate readers, helping yourself, your loved ones, your communities, and the world become a better place.

APPROBATION FOR SOULFIT, BY YITZHAK AFTALION

Four years ago, a young man attended our summer personal growth program (STEP). My first impression was that emotional and spiritual growth was important to him (why else attend the program?), but they would not be the center of his life over the long haul. We parted ways at the end of the summer, and I expected him to go his own way and be successful in life, but not to write books on personal growth. Alas, we all make mistakes in our thoughts about people.

Over the coming years, I received many emails from him about his involvement in various projects to help others reach their full potential. Then, to an even greater surprise, our young man, Yitzhak Aftalion, informed me he had put all his experience and ideas together into a personal growth book, Soulfit.

He has created a fascinating fusion of personal experience, modern-day science/medicine, and ancient wisdom to produce something that is both enlightening and practical and inspiring. We live in a society that values physical beauty and physical abilities. Still, he shows convincingly that a person can never reach their full potential without attention to emotional and spiritual aspects.

He shows this from his experience in professional sports and

Examples taken from the coaches of some legendary basketball dynasties. Speaking of coaches, the author himself speaks to you from the pages like a caring, passionate coach who knows how to motivate and inspire. He wants you to succeed in the ultimate game of life. Read this book and reread it to absorb the eternal life lessons that it contains.

Yonasan Sigler

Director, STEP Jerusalem (www.step.org.il)

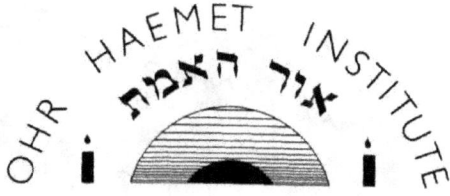

OHR HAEMET INSTITUTE / אור האמת

Rabbi E. Ben-David *zz"l*
Founder

Rabbi D. Akhamzadeh
Director

Rabbi Y. Govhari
Rosh Kellel

Rabbi Y. Mahtov
Assistant Director

July 20 2020

To whom it may concern:

My good friend, Mr. Yitzchak A has authored a book named Soulfit. I leafed through the book and found it full of sound advice on healthy living habits for body and soul. These advices are results of his research and investigation over the years and referenced by their sources in our Holy writings.

This book stems from Yitzchak's good heart and desire to help others and share his knowledge and findings with all.

I bless him in this and all his future endeavors with Divine help and success.

Rabbi David M. Akhamzdeh

Director

בס"ד

הרב אלון גוונ לא שלום וברכה,

אליך גוונה באוה החתן זהן לאהן רב גולה
ונהיה נסתרי, הב .בחה. וכן ולאן הנהרנ ין
כי, באלה .וכן ולהשאן הבן אלה שבה ספר וקהשי
וכן אחה .אלאאנה רבה רבאה אלק קלדל קולאאן גוני
ולקרהאהה .רחה הלההיה .את לקרדל את רח אלאהנה ולן
ולדאהה .ולאשנה הבה באהונה ורבלון אלאהנאה

ולקהלן ולקאן רב.אן .ף.אן .ל.אני .ובון .פלבי .הר
הר אל.ה .ואן .וחולי .י רב .הקה. הבקה בסה אלאן
וקן .אלאה סבה לורב לוי ן .לדה אחה .הבקה .וי חול
.לולה .ולאהת הרביה. לקבלה את רב. ולה. אן
את בשאלוו ולבוה גון .רחאלה .ורבון .ראון
רבה .רבה .ולאן שון ורנ. שלן רבאהה רבה
לאנוו יהלן :שאלה .שלאה רבבה
נוגן.

Table of Contents

LET'S START

PROFESSIONAL SPORT, SOCIETY, PHONES, AND MOVIES

Our world has changed drastically, and it is evident in today's world. Our media seems to be misinforming and confusing our society with an overall lack of political leadership. Our focus in this book will be to try to deliver real, raw truths and also to inspire with divine information to help us all make better decisions. We will start by speaking about today's sports world, professional athletes, our society's challenges, and more.

In today's professional sports, marketing and money have taken over. For instance, many players earn millions of dollars in today's business-savvy world before they even reach the court/field, regardless of their own court/field performances. Contracts and deals are being thrown at kids and their families from high school levels, sometimes even in youth leagues.

This, without a doubt, can inhibit the competitive spirit of the players, as they are assured of excellent financial results, irrespective of the quality of their sporting performances. Because we have replaced true efforts and rewards with the craze for only earning colossal salaries and developing a marketing brand for each major athlete, such a preoccupation with material gains can damage the before-earning. This dramatic reward can damage the inner psyche of a player and the people around them if not filtered properly. Take it from someone who has seen players and clients alike become affected. Just look at the stats. Those who have won the lottery often end up bankrupt with worse lives.

Many times, it is a curse more than a blessing. Getting things without earning them can lead to ungratefulness and foolishness. It cannot be emphasized enough that there is a dangerous pattern to receiving things, particularly monetary awards, too quickly or, in our case, athletes getting too much money early on, which cannot only cheapen motivation and hence the game or championship but can ultimately ruin a player's life. It is foolish to take the eyes off the ball as a fellow team member to pursue personal fame, wealth, and glory instead.

First, it leads to instant gratification, the desire to experience pleasure or fulfillment without delay or deferment. Whatever you want, you want it now. Instant gratification is the opposite of what we have been taught, and we try hard to practice delayed gratification. I have seen this for myself, and when training with NBA players. Many of them get huge contracts before earning them. This leads to an inflated ego and a dangerous attitude of wanting things right away.

Not all, but many of these players are a burden off the court, negatively affecting teams. Do not get me wrong, many have a fantastic work ethic, drive, and God-given talents. However, with off-court temptations and life decisions, many make terrible choices. I have seen players blow money on their lusts and desires, and for the family, it is a catastrophe filled with lies.

Everyone wants to be a father and mother, but the way many of these players take on these roles is quite sad. According to statistics, the divorce rate among all professional athletes is between 60% and 80%, according to the New York Times and Sports Illustrated, which is higher than the average American divorce rate of 50%. Besides infidelity and issues dealing with money, fame, and travel, they have drastic effects.

These players need help, and many of them do not have the tools. Today's athletes are not the same role models we once had in the 90s, 80s, and 70s, who were great to many of us growing up. For instance, the ESPN documentary "Broke" states, "By the time they have been retired for two years, 78% of former NFL players have gone bankrupt or are under financial stress." Many of these athletes, whom I have met personally, are good-hearted people. But in today's world, being goodhearted is not enough. One needs to be educated on financial responsibility (saving and spending, etc.) and the discipline of delayed gratification, not to mention doing some soul searching. Athletes need to examine deep down inside and look at their long-term goals to see what they want from life. We are all here for a limited amount of time. So why not learn and explore the meaning behind life? How did we get here? Where are we going next? What is the point of existence? What do I want to leave behind? A lot of education needs to be put in place.

We hope to educate people so they can also educate others. Ethical old-fashioned commitment, necessary life skills, and sacrifice seem like lost arts to this new generation of athletes. There is indeed a lot to learn from sports, such as preparation and hard work.

"You can't have confidence unless you are prepared. Failure to prepare is preparing to fail. There is no substitute for hard work. If you're looking for an easy way or a trick, it might work for a while, but you will not develop the talents that lie within you. There is simply no substitute for work." John Wooden (coach with the most victories in college sports history). We can take the good and learn from everything. First, however, we must be honest that sports and society are not what they used to be and can pose more harm than good to our spiritual goals and family values.

Phones

A Nielsen Company study shows that the average American spends a staggering 11 hours and 54 minutes each day connected to some form of media: TV, smartphones, radio, or games. That is up nearly an hour and a half in only a year. Moreover, smartphone usage accounts for virtually all the increases. For example, people spent just under four hours a day on their phones in Nielsen's most recent study, compared to 2 hours and 31 minutes in the final three months of 2018.

A walk through the train on a daily commute shows how absorbed people are in their phones, and they are becoming increasingly comfortable using them to watch videos. As noted in the study, "They are finding more and more ways to keep their attention occupied."

Another study shows that the average adult may spend the equivalent of 34 years of their lives staring at screens, according to a poll! A questionnaire taken by 2,000 people in Britain found that they spent over 4,866 hours a year on average using gadgets such as phones, laptops, and televisions. This works out to 301,733 hours over the average adult lifetime of 62 years. Three and a half hours a day were spent looking at TV screens, at least four hours staring at laptops, and two hours on mobile phones. Also, people said they thought less than half the time they spent on these devices was "productive."

We note that the use of smartphones helps save time with shopping, banking, and paying bills, and of course, sending essential lessons and messages to friends and family. If we only used the phone for these purposes, it would be great. But the problem is that this gift can be a curse if not taken care of. The problem lies in the games, movies, and addictions the phone brings that can waste our valuable time, beam unnecessary radio waves into the body and brain, and perhaps damage our beloved relationships and family life.

I mean, it is obvious how you can ask kids to stop using their phones if the adults are always using them. We will talk more about this later on. First, however, it is essential to be aware of the stats and where we are headed as a society. We suggest giving yourself and the phone a break and tapping more into your relationships, learning, exercising, working, and more.

There are so many natural ways to spend time with ourselves and our loved ones. Therefore, we should consider these statistics and try to make meaningful lifestyle changes. Please note that thoughts made about sports, movies, or any other mundane topics are intended for those with challenges in these areas. We have separated the citations purposefully to distinguish (in Hebrew, we say lehavdíl) the mundane from holy topics.

Movies today are just not the same as they used to be. Instead, violence, nudity, and other cheap thrills are occupying our time and minds.

We can see that the same types of films from the 50s, 60s, and even the 80s are different. From modesty in dressing to family values, things have changed drastically since the year 2000.

Many good family values are absent from what Hollywood is showing. We will later discuss this in greater detail, but the point is to show it is time you become the real star of your own "movie" and stop looking for role models in today's movies.

ROADMAP:
METHODOLOGY OF THE PROGRAM

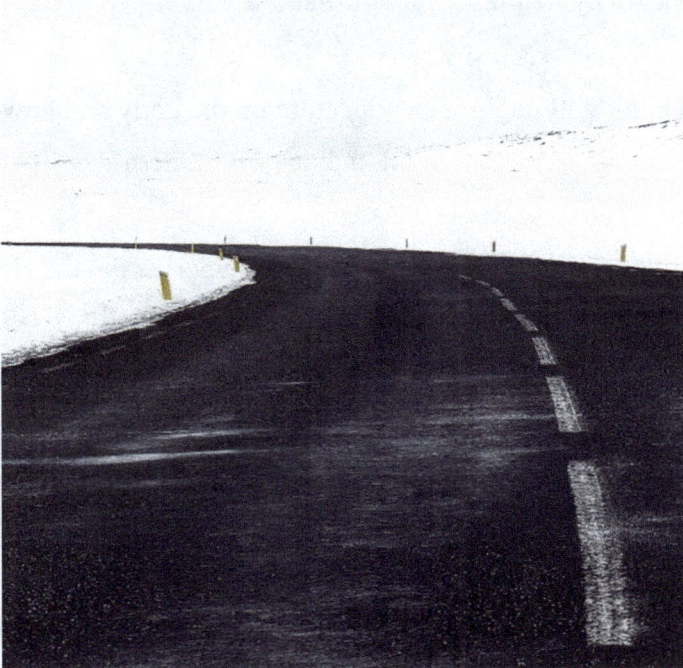

Many people get sidetracked when they read diet, fitness, or spiritual books, so we changed that in Soulfit by ensuring you envision and prepare your game plan. Then, as you read and practice the material, tools, and exercises, take notes along the journey. Here are a few tips to help you maximize this experience and remember what you are learning: Clear your mind of all judgments; start this process with a blank canvas.

Like an empty glass, you must be clear to pour in the water (information). But please remember that you can only pour water from your glass for those looking to become coaches or help others.

Help others only when your glass is appropriately full. So, start empty and begin by helping yourself first.

This book will begin with education on the body and how food affects us. It will then transition into advice for modern-day life and draw out the connection with our Master.

Keep in mind to try your best to memorize the mission statement, the most important quote of the book, and Rambam's "Four Fundamental Rules" (Body Section #10). Get them down cold. Try them out and keep them in mind when you go to the market, a restaurant, or even cook at home. Then we will explain the importance of exercising your body and your mind as well. The power of the mind is a crucial section; review it many times. Make it a habit. At any point, use our website (soulfit.com) as a reference point. Each student has their path to follow.

Please remember to find a type of exercise that you enjoy. You will do more for your fitness when doing things you enjoy. We also include recovery techniques that are essential to recharging, so you can keep striving forward. Practice these recovery techniques whenever the information becomes too heavy.

After the Body and Mind Section, we will delve into perhaps the deepest part of the book, which for many will be the most difficult the Soul Section.

Remember, our spiritual journey is not "all or nothing." It takes time, and everyone's task is unique. In other words, do not compare yourself to others. We may be part of a collective soul, but GOD has created us to be individually unique.

"If I am I because I am I, and you are you because you are you, then I am I, and you are you. But if I am I because you are you and you are you because I am I, then I am not I, and you are not you."

Rabbi Menachem Mendel Morgensztern of Kotzk,
known as the Kotzker Rebbe

As you read and practice the materials, techniques, and exercises, it is advisable to take notes. Applying this book's principles may change your perspective about trials and hard times, thus helping to set you on the path to wellness and greatness.
With Soulfit, you will get timeless information for your mind, body, and soul. Therefore, we urge you to train now and be prepared for life.

Life is truly a rollercoaster for everybody (not just you and me), and you certainly will have to do some uphill climbing. The key is to take all negative hits gracefully, figure out how to turn them into positives, and keep moving forward. That is how, with GOD's help, you will win. Remember to remain grateful each day and keep your expectations in check; working hard and expecting little is a great recipe for feeling happy.

Also, just like your favorite dance move or jump shot, you have to keep practicing to keep it sharp and on point. Finally, keep your feet nimble and your movements artistic. Successful people never stop learning throughout life.

Final point

You do not need palm readers, gurus, astrologers, or fortune tellers to help you find the energy or make your life decisions. This book aims to guide and help you discover the answers to questions that plague your mind. You have all the answers inside of you. All you need is help to break down the husks of impurities built inside to understand your essence.

In addition, many people are getting several kinds of cleanses in their bodies, but you have to start with your mind, body, and soul. Begin with small steps, and at your own pace. Soon enough, you will conquer your mountain and, with Hashem's help, have your own redemption.

SECTION I

THE BODY

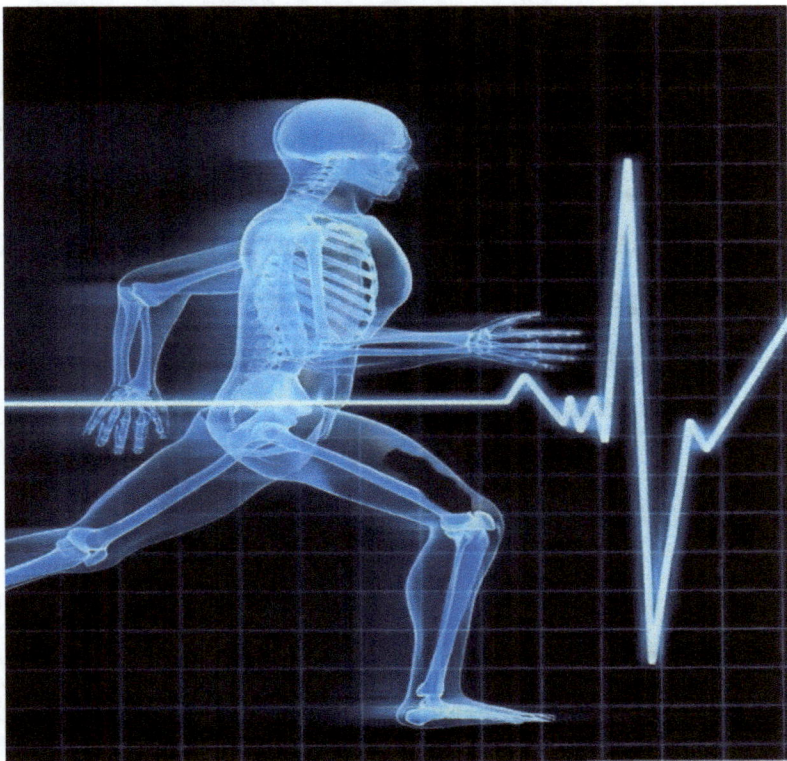

The following is our #1 goal for the Soulfit Training Program, as well as our mission statement:

"Get your body strong and your mind focused
So you can better serve your soul!"

When I was preparing to go overseas for basketball, I was introduced to a nutrition teacher and coach. His name was Coach Wayne Douglas, the founder of Elite Health Food. I would like to share here, but first, a quick bio. Coach Wayne began working as a high school biology and chemistry teacher in the Los Angeles area. While teaching high school students, he spent his free time designing nutrition and supplementation programs for high-caliber athletes. His clients ranged from Olympic athletes to professional football, basketball, and baseball players, as well as college athletes at universities across the United States.

1) Food Fundamentals

Why should we give any attention to the way we combine the various foods we eat? Why shouldn't we eat what we want whenever we please? The answer to these questions is quite simple. Our digestive tracts are not designed to digest complex foods that we combine without discretion.

There are many important reasons for combining our foods correctly. Before the nutrients from the foods we eat can be absorbed through the intestinal tract and transported to the cells of our body (via the bloodstream), they must first be broken down into simpler biochemical formations. The key components necessary for this process are called enzymes.

Enzymes are the active elements in digestive liquids responsible for our food's proper chemical breakdown and digestion. These enzymes have unique functions and definite limits in their capabilities. Different digestive enzymes are secreted for digesting specific types of food. For example, the enzyme that helps digest fats will not break down protein or carbohydrates.

Likewise, the enzyme that digests carbohydrates will not work on fats or proteins. Likewise, the body's process for the digestion of proteins differs from the process used to digest carbohydrates and starches. Yet, through a divine master plan, they can all work simultaneously.

Understanding that our digestive enzymes have particular functions and biochemical limitations clarifies that our systems were not designed to simultaneously digest many types of foods. As a result, poorly digested foods produce toxic metabolic byproducts. The buildup of these toxins in the body (called mucoid plaque) can be the source of many serious health problems.

Although changing our dietary habits can present a challenge, the rewards of vitality and improvements in health and well-being are worth the effort. There are remarkable benefits to be gained—physically, emotionally, mentally, and spiritually—when we cooperate with our bodies' biological capabilities and follow the principles of the right food combinations.

2) Mucoid Plaque

Mucoid plaque is a substance that can gradually build up in the body because of poorly digested food. This mass of toxic, mucus-like matter protects the body from unhealthy foods, stress, drugs, pesticides, etc. Mucoid plaque accumulates until it is several inches thick and may reach the entire length of the stomach, small intestines, and colon.

While this layer of plaque protects the body from particular harmful food substances, it can also prevent the body from adequately assimilating vitamins, minerals, and food nutrients. Autopsies have revealed colons measuring up to 18 inches in diameter because they were packed with layers of this encrusted mucoid fecal matter, some weighing up to forty pounds.

3) Symptoms of Poor Digestion

- Constipation
- Intestinal Gas
- Diarrhea
- Muscle Soreness
- Bone Soreness

- Mucus
- Headaches
- Anxiety
- Insomnia
- Skin breakouts (i.e., psoriasis, acne, etc.)
- Bad breath.
- Yeast infection (most of the time leading to a white coating on the tongue)
- Dry hair, Fatigue, Bloating

4) Proteins

Proteins are one of the most abundant substances in the body. They are used to build and repair tissue and are essential in keeping good health and vitality. Proteins are composed of smaller substances called amino acids and are more complex than fats or carbohydrates. They are digested through the proteolytic (protein-splitting) enzymes: pepsin and trypsin. Protein requires an acidic medium in which to digest. Therefore, protein-rich foods and starchy carbohydrate-rich foods (which require an alkaline medium for digestion) should be eaten at separate meals. Fats slow the digestive process, so it is better not to combine fats and protein simultaneously.

Due to how quickly they digest simple sugars (fruits, honey, syrups, etc.), they should not be eaten with protein, which requires a more complex and prolonged process. "Meat consumption in the United States has nearly doubled in the last century. Americans are now among the top per capita meat consumers in the world.

The average American eats over three times the global average."
A good number of researchers have shown that "Americans' taste for meat and animal products is putting them at higher risk for a range of health problems." The best high-quality protein sources will be found in fresh fruit, vegetables, raw nuts and seeds, whole grains, and legumes.

Now, we are not saying to completely get rid of all meat and poultry. We are simply suggesting being aware and finding a balance of nutrition that is right for you.

5) Carbohydrates

Carbohydrates are the primary source of energy for all bodily functions. They provide us with calories that are readily available for the body to use as energy. Carbohydrates are often referred to as sugars or starches. We should get these mainly from fruits, vegetables, seeds, nuts, and whole-grain cereals (complex carbohydrates).

The body converts all sugars and starches into simple sugars, such as glucose (for immediate use by the body) or glycogen (stored for energy). These simple sugars are used as fuel for the muscular and nervous systems and the brain. Simple sugars, such as those found in honey and fruit, are easily digested. Starches such as those found in whole grains are more complex. These complex carbs eventually get broken down into glucose. Cellulose, a carbohydrate found in the skin and fiber of fruits and vegetables, supplies bulk for useful intestinal functions and proper elimination.

Elimination is a critical sign that things are functioning properly[1] within our bodies. A few days without excretion means you need to work on your fiber intake and change your eating patterns. The main Enzymes involved in carbohydrate/starch digestion are salivary. Amylase (called ptyalin) and pancreatic amylase (called amylopsin).

Carbohydrates, such as rich starchy foods, require an alkaline medium for proper digestion. Therefore, eat such foods at separate meal times when consuming protein-rich foods (which require an acidic medium for digestion). In addition, since sugars such as fruits are so quickly digested, avoid eating them in combination with complex carbohydrates (grains, bread, potatoes), which require a more complex and prolonged digestive process.
Consumption of "refined" carbohydrate foods, such as white flour products, white sugar, candy, sodas, and other junk foods, can cause toxicity and vitamin and mineral deficiencies in the body, leading to serious health problems.

6) Fats

Fats, also called lipids, are the most concentrated source of energy in the diet. They are compounds forming carbon, hydrogen, and oxygen, the same elements found in carbohydrates, but present in

_____

different combinations and proportions.

Besides supplying energy, fats serve as carriers for fat-soluble vitamins (A, D, E, and K). Thus, fats are an integral part of the process whereby calcium is made available to the body's tissues. They are also crucial for helping the body convert carotene to vitamin A under the influence of lipases (fat-splitting enzymes) secreted by the pancreas. Fats and oils are broken down into glycerol and fatty acids. Fatty acids are necessary for normal growth and healthy blood, arteries, and nerves. Glycerol is converted (in the liver) into glucose or glycogen to fuel energy. Oils are like fats but are usually liquid at room temperature. Fats and oils slow down and inhibit digestion. Therefore, it is best to avoid eating fats and protein at the same meal.

Fats derived from animal sources have been linked to many health problems. The highest quality sources of fats and oils are fresh fruits such as avocados, olives, raw nuts, seeds, whole grains, and legumes. A good sample plate for good fats and proteins would be freshly cooked fish (salmon, tuna) with a side salad including avocado and olives.

7) Two-Sample Recipes

Champion Stew

Bring 1520 cups of water to a boil. Add a package of fresh mixed vegetables you like, assuming they are ready (add a package of cut corn if you like it). If frozen, please prepare it first with water only.

Once ready:

- Add a packet of green beans.
- Add generous chunks of ready chicken breast and turkey breast, cut into pieces of chicken.
- Season with onion powder, garlic powder, cayenne, and turmeric.
- Do not add any beans, rice, pasta, or potatoes. Let it simmer, and when ready, serve.

Power Sandwich

Start with low-carbohydrate bread, sprouted bread, or seven- or eight-grain bread. You can also use low-carb tortillas to make wraps if you prefer. Add:

- Mustard
- Lettuce or spinach
- Sliced red onion
- Sliced cucumber
- Sliced squash
- Meat choice (either chicken or turkey)
- Grated carrots
- Alfalfa sprouts or other sprouts (wash first)

8) Modern-Day Nutritional Advice

- Do not eat when emotionally upset, stressed, or directly after a hard workout.

- Eat only when hungry and stop before you are full.
- Do not eat foods that are too hot or too cold; they can damage the enzymes necessary for proper digestion. The room temperature is the best.
- Always avoid refined, canned, fried, and processed foods
- Learning to combine foods properly is not just a passing trend. The principles of proper food combining are scientific, biochemical facts of life
- Health is wealth! I cannot emphasize this enough. If we do not have our health, nothing else is ever going to matter
- A positive and loving attitude toward yourself, others, and life, along with a healthy diet, ultimately means a long, joyous, and productive life!

When you are ready to progress to the next level, we will take this information and unite it with ancient knowledge. You will see how much of our current scientific understanding is rooted in ancient texts, such as Maimonides' Mishneh Torah. Modern will meet ancient, giving you information to empower yourself to build a better diet and cultivate more healthful exercise habits.

9) Maimonides (The Rambam)

Rabbi Moshe ben Maimon, Talmudist, Halachist, physician, and communal leader, known in the Jewish world by the acronym "Rambam" and the world at large as "Maimonides," is one of the most influential figures in the history of Torah scholarship. Today, many hospitals and schools across the globe are named after Maimonides, and to this day, students worldwide are.

Pore over his scholarly works. We will attempt to connect ancient to modern-day wisdom on wellness and spirituality.

10) Ancient/Timeless Health Principles

Modern-day science is continually discovering new fruits and plants, and with technological advances, we can learn and uncover more than the earlier generations. However, the key is to understand that just because technology changes does not mean everything else must change as well. Yes, certain things will change, but other things will not. We are at a crucial point in human history and need to understand where we came from and where we are going. What is the significance of this food?

In each generation, extremely beneficial herbs and fruits were discovered unknown to earlier generations. The human mind cannot grasp all the advantages of each plant, but their benefits will become known through scientific experiments in times to come, as so many already have[2].

Rambam reasons that including health rules in a person's daily regimen is necessary for a healthy body and essential to serve GOD properly. He further adds that it is ultimately impossible to understand anything of GOD in depth when one is ill. Therefore, we must avoid

---

anything detrimental to our health and focus on activities that promote a healthy mind and body.

According to the Rambam, the recipe for achieving optimum health includes four major principles:

1. A person who exercises and exerts himself powerfully, does not satiate himself, and has loose bowels will probably not become ill, and his strength will increase, even if he eats bad food.

2. A person who does not exercise, delays relieving himself, or has constipation will suffer from pain all his life, and his strength will fade even if the right foods are eaten and all the rules of medicine are kept.

3. Overeating is like poison to the body and is the leading cause of all illnesses.

Unhealthy foods cause most illnesses, or by gorging oneself, even with healthy eating!

In short, the four key ingredients for achieving optimum physical health, in order of importance, are:

1. Food Quantity
2. Exercise
3. Food Quality
4. Waste Management

After you learn the above principles, you will put yourself in the best possible position to achieve your fitness and nutrition goals.

We want you to succeed beyond that! We will share more information that is rarely discussed. However, the secret to achieving your goals in this world includes physical and spiritual health (inextricably connected to your mind and body). A holistic approach that treats the body as one organism is the key to success. The Rambam's principles are an essential piece of the Soulfit program.

Now, let us delve a little deeper into each of these four items so that we can understand more precisely how to apply them to our daily life needs:

11) Food Quantity

Of the four guidelines, the most critical tool in Rambam's protocol is knowing how much and when to eat. You should not eat until you have made sure you do not need to relieve yourself. (See more in the section on waste management below.) Also, you should not eat until you have taken a stroll at a sufficient pace to raise your body temperature (see more about body temperature below).

Eat until you are 75% full. Stop eating when you feel the satisfaction of a full stomach. Maimonides teaches that eating the proper amount is the most helpful to heal the damage to your digestive tract. We understand we are not meant to pack our stomachs. We have a natural digestive system that has been designed to do its job, and it is a particular size for a reason. We must never overload it.

You do not need to drink very much during a meal. As said, our

Bodies have natural enzymes that help us digest food, and we do not need to oversaturate them. If you must drink, it is okay to drink only a small amount of water during the meal.

If you do not like water with food, it is wise to have a little wine (at night); of course, only a cup or less. If the wine is too strong, one can mix it with some water. Wine (in responsible and minimal amounts) is very healthful and can benefit digestion and circulation, and the increase in antioxidants is also good for the heart. (Please note that wine is not as beneficial for minors as it is for adults.)

12) Exercise

Being overweight is dangerous physically, emotionally, and even spiritually. People who do not exercise will probably suffer from pain and depleted energy levels even if they eat the right foods and follow all the medical rules.[3] You should not eat until you have walked enough to warm your body or done some work or exercise (preferably in the morning) before a meal. Ideally, exert yourself to the point of working up a sweat each morning.

Afterward, you should briefly rest until you recover and then eat. If a person bathes in hot water after exerting himself, it would also be beneficial to slow down the heart rate, calm the muscles, and relax.

---

the body. Afterward, *"he should wait a short while to eat."*[4] Exercising is a cornerstone of health, and in our program as well. It keeps the lungs and heart active while also strengthening muscles and even helping to improve moods. It is preferable to exercise in the early morning and before food (not after).

Rambam says that anyone who takes a stroll or exerts himself after eating can bring severe and harmful illnesses upon himself. Ancient physicians wrote about the three major components of an exercise program: cardio, strengthening, and stretching. These concepts are still relevant today. We encourage you to find an activity you enjoy most and try to participate in it for at least thirty to forty minutes each day.

Examples of suitable activities include walking, jogging, running, hiking, basketball, tennis, soccer, dancing, etc. The best type of exercise influences the soul positively and causes it to rejoice or energize you! For instance, if you like to hike, then hike as your workout. If you want to swim, swim. If you wish to shoot some hoops, then ball! Do what you are naturally inclined to do for fun.

Staying active will keep you in shape longer, and you will also improve at your chosen sport or activity. Remember, the minimum is about twenty minutes a day, roughly four to five times per week, depending on your age and weight. Adding more is better, but keep in mind that you do not want to overdo it. You do not want

---

To deplete your muscles and body and overexert yourself. Just keep it simple to achieve optimal form.

Exercise is fundamental to our health, and sometimes we must push ourselves. Like all things, there will be days when you feel more tired or less motivated, but I can assure you, once you tie up those kicks and get on that bicycle, field, court, treadmill, or whatever you do, you will have taken the first steps toward a new you! Once you get going, you will feel much better.

You will increase blood flow in your body. Exercising muscles need more blood. And in response to regular exercise, they actually grow more blood vessels by expanding the network of capillaries. In turn, muscle cells boost levels of the enzymes that allow them to use oxygen to generate energy. The small steps create a solid foundation for building a new life and a brand-new destiny for you.

13) Food Quality

The following two sections are secondary principles. First, take a backseat to exercise and food quantity. In Maimonides' days, they did not have conveniences such as refrigeration and processing, as we have today. So, of course, they ate more natural, organic, and fresher foods. It is only logical that the sooner you eat the food, once it comes off that tree or out of the ground, the more nutrients you are going to get. Try to shop at the most farm-direct places you can (i.e., a farmers' market).

However, be sure not to forget the most essential point of the food quantity section above. Even if you fill your belly with the freshest foods, it can still be extremely harmful because our digestive tracts are not meant for that type of abuse. The Rambam also allows for the "sweet tooth" (ice cream, pastries, cakes, candies, etc.), as long as you never stuff yourself. A tasty dessert is perfectly fine after a meal. For example, eat your appetizer and full-course meal until you are nearly full (a little less than 75%), and leave enough room for dessert.

This way, you will help your system do its job, and you will be happy at the same time. WINWIN.

14) Waste Management

You should never put off relieving yourself, even for an instant. Instead, whenever the need to urinate or defecate arises, do so at once. When one is constipated, it is a sign that illness is approaching. If you are healthy internally, you will not usually experience problems with waste management.

Maimonides also says that one should not pray or communicate with GOD if one has the urge to use the restroom. This waste waiting to leave the body makes a person impure, so they must wash their hands and even say words of prayer after using the restroom to get back to a state of purity.

15) Tips and Insights

Patience, education, and that neuron-changing attitude of "practice makes perfect" will lead you to better habits. In time, you will see a positive transformation towards a better you.

We highly recommend that you review and practice the four principles from the earlier chapter until they become a habit. In this section, we will give some additional tips. Although they are secondary to the four major principles, they are vital. A few details on eating properly:
Rambam states we should always eat... while reclining on our side. It was customary for men of importance to recline on couches in Talmudic times, as in Greek and Roman circles. The advice to favor the left side is from Pesach. The reason is that the food may enter the windpipe rather than the gullet and cause the person to (heaven forbid) choke.

16) Sleep Insights

Day and night make up twenty-four hours. It is sufficient for humans to sleep one-third of this period. Eight hours. Preferably from the beginning of his sleep to sunrise. Thus, you should ideally rise from your bed. The Rambam advises pre-sunrise awakening to allow
time to recite morning prayers and the Shema for Jews. However, even for Gentiles or Noahides, it is rewarding to wake up pre-sunrise and thank the Creator. Yes, He understands your heart and all languages. Highly successful people wake up early and retire early (wise men as

well, as the saying goes).

You should not sleep face down or on your back. Instead, you should lie on your left and then your right side by the end of the night. You should not retire shortly after eating but should wait three to four hours.

To sleep more efficiently, eating an early dinner will give you enough time to digest your food. Rambam suggests one should strive to sleep at 10 PM and rise at 6 AM (depending on sunrise). However, this may vary depending on the season. Yalkut Yosef (edition 5764, vol. 1, pg. 64) writes that it is unhealthy to sleep more than 8 or less than 6 hours; it all depends on the health and age of the person.

17) Food Insights

Laxative foods, such as grapes, figs, mulberries, pears, and melons, should be eaten before a meal. However, one should not consume them with the main meal. Instead, one should wait until they have descended from the upper stomach and eat their meal (this is roughly thirty minutes)

18) Meat

A person who desires to eat poultry and meat in one sitting should eat the poultry first. Similarly, if they wish to eat both eggs and poultry, they should eat the eggs first. Furthermore, if one desires to eat both the meat of large cattle (bovine family) and that of small cattle (ovine family), one should eat the meat of the small cattle first. They should always eat the lighter fare first and the heavier afterward.

19) Body Temperature

Rambam speaks of body temperature as an essential point. This is not one of his primary principles, but it is still an important one. One should try to keep one's body temperature balanced. Everyone has a somewhat different body temperature. This natural variation is why friends or family can drive us crazy (with the heater or A/C).

The Chinese dietary principle of Yin and Yang (derived from these teachings) is a concept that stresses the importance of balance, just as Rambam always did in his theory. When the weather is warm, one should eat cold and uncooked foods and vice versa.

The same principle also applies to bland and well-spiced foods when the weather is cold. One should warm oneself with spiced foods, whereas when it is hot out, one should refrain from spices to prevent exhaustion and overheating.

20) Cooling Foods

Depending on what part of the globe you live in, it is beneficial to cool the body during summer or warmer climates. One way to do this, according to Maimonides, is to eat foods that do not have many spices. Another critical item to help cool the body is vinegar. Rambam notes that vinegar acts to avert gases and diarrhea (Regimen of Health, 4:14).

These attributes make it a desirable ingredient in food during hot weather when there is a risk of dehydration.

Shabbat 113b quotes from the book of Ruth (2:14), "As the righteous Ruth of Moab was working in the desert heat, overexerting herself in the fields of Boaz, the verse states...and you will dip your bread in the vinegar." This quote proves that vinegar was a valuable part of the diet in extreme heat during biblical times.

Besides vinegar, another option to cool your body and get you back on an even keel in the heat can be watermelon. Watermelon comprises 90% water, which helps keep people well hydrated.

Also, watermelon contains loads of vitamins A and C, has no fat, and is packed with lycopene, an antioxidant that may aid in the prevention of cancer and cardiovascular disease. Other good cooling foods include cucumbers, radishes, and even mint. These can help replenish and cool the body.

21) Chilled Out Salad

- Toss pieces of cucumber and radishes
- A drizzle of olive oil and balsamic vinegar
- A sprinkle of fresh mint (wash properly, remove dirt and bugs) leaves or kale for a heat-blasting salad to keep you chill in the tropical heat.

Drinks

Many of today's sports beverages (with sodium and sugar) can make your dehydration worse. In addition, frozen foods and drinks (like ice cream) can interfere with digestion and the body's need to sweat as a natural cooling mechanism. So, however tempting it may be to sit on your porch, licking an ice cream cone to beat the heat, opt for a wedge of watermelon or other types of melon.

Perhaps reconsider Gatorade (with all the sugar). Instead, we recommend our Mintyrade or Vita Mint. It is lemonade from Israel, but I add coconut water. For hydration, try fresh coconut water; no added sugar is needed. All that is required is water, or if need be, throw some mint leaves in there. There is a new trend in using an infuser pitcher for your water. Just add cucumber and mint to the filter for a refreshing, flavorful beverage. The Rambam Protocol can help save you and your summer!

22) Warming Foods

In the winter or rainy season, you should eat seasoned foods. Also, use many spices (turmeric) and condiments like mustard and chiltit (an aromatic herb scientifically known as In other parts of the world, it is known by names such as asasant, food of GOD, jowani badian, stinking gum, or ting.

Asafoetida was described by Arab and Islamic scientists and pharmacists, such as Ibn al-Baitar and Fakhr al-Din al-Razi, as having some positive medicinal effects on the respiratory system. After the Roman Empire fell, until the 16th century, asafoetida (fennel family) was rare in Europe, and it was viewed as a medicinal substance rather than an herb.

Other foods that can help to warm us up are oatmeal, lean meats, and almonds. Soups are also helpful, especially black bean and pumpkin. However, if you just want what the Rambam ordered, check out the green dish in the next section.

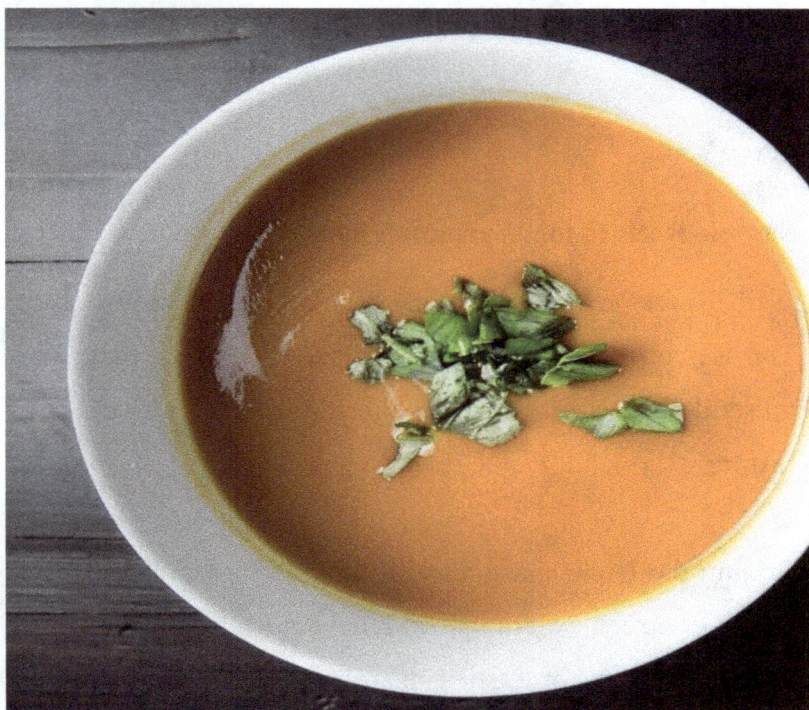

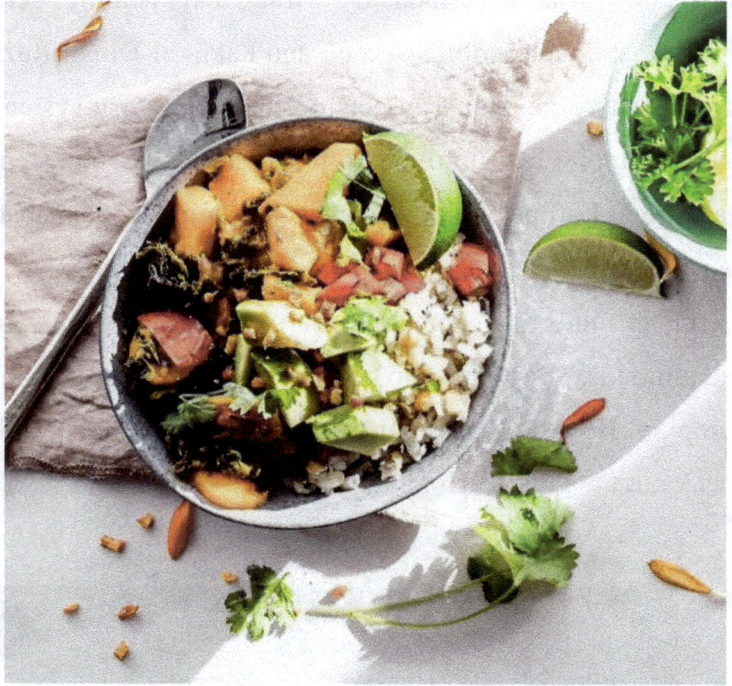

Sample Recipes for Warming Foods:

This recipe uses spices that Maimonides recommends for winter. The asafoetida is sautéed with garlic to mellow the pungency, and the mustard seed is toasted with sliced almonds to give a nice roasted texture.

Adding the Dijon mustard will ultimately provide this dish with its 'kick'—you can experiment with how much to add. Add more to ramp up the spice level or less if you are cooking for milder palates.

Ingredients

- 1 Head of lettuce or cabbage, or the like
- ½ cup sliced raw almonds
- 1 Garlic clove, minced
- 1 Tablespoon olive oil
- 1 Tablespoon mustard seed
- ½ Teaspoon asafoetida powder
- 12 teaspoons of Dijon mustard mixed with one tablespoon of water, salt, and freshly ground black pepper.

Heat a dry skillet over medium-high heat.

Add the mustard seed and almonds and continually shake the skillet until the fragrant aromas are released and the mustard pops (around 35 minutes).

Now pour the oil into the pan, along with the garlic and asafetida. With a wooden spoon, sauté for about 90 seconds until the garlic is golden. Add the greens and toss to coat them with the oil combination in the pan. Season with salt and pepper to taste; add the Dijon/water mixture.

Cover the pan and cook on low heat for three minutes. Uncover, toss with toasted almonds/mustard, and enjoy!

23) Other worthy tips

- Here are a few more random points from Maimonides that I would like to add here: Honey and wine are harmful to the young and wholesome for older adults, especially those 50 and over.
- The older one gets, the better wine and honey are for one's health.
- Indeed, more wine and honey are needed in the rainy and winter seasons. The body is less active and usually in colder temperatures; wine can balance your temperature, help circulation, and more, as we have said earlier.
- In summer, one should eat two-thirds of what one eats in winter to aid heat and digestion. Whoever conducts himself in the ways we have outlined in this section, the Rambam guarantees them:
  - They will not become idle.
  - They will not need a doctor.
  - Their bodies will remain intact.

In addition, Rambam says that one may rely on this guarantee unless their body has been impaired from birth, they were accustomed to one of the harmful habits from birth, or there is a plague or drought in the world.

All these beneficial habits apply only to individuals who are ready to quit their dangerous lifestyles. Suppose one, however, has a diseased organ or has fallen ill because of a harmful lifestyle. In that case, each of these must choose distinct patterns of behavior following his particular illness, as is explained in Maimonides's medical literature.

Similarly, individuals with character disorders should ideally be ready to give up their habits. Otherwise, these principles will not work for them. Instead, they should seek an expert who will direct them to correct their faults.

- In a city where there is no doctor available, neither the healthy nor the sick man should budge from adhering to all the directions given by Maimonides, for each of them ultimately brings benefit.

- A sick person should ideally have a more personalized program for their health, but if that is not available, they should follow Rambam's general rules, for they will, as we said, bring about a state of health.

- A Torah sage may not live in a community that does not have the following: a doctor, a bloodletter, a bathhouse, a restroom, an available water source (river or spring) for Jews, a synagogue, a teacher of children, a scribe, a charity supervisor, and a rabbinical court empowered to impose corporal punishment and jail sentences.

- The merit of the Torah study of young children maintained the world. Accordingly, a city that does not hire a person to teach its children the Torah may be ostracized by others and even destroyed.

The Rambam advises us, "Just as the wise man is recognized through his wisdom and his temperaments, and in these, he stands apart from the rest of the people, he should be recognized through his actions—in his eating, drinking, sexual relations, and in relieving himself." These actions should be exceptionally becoming and befitting.

24) Intimate Relations

From a women's class via

https://torah.org/learning/womenclass3/

"The Western world, the culture we live in, has considerable difficulty with the concept of sexual intimacy. One indication is the culture's obsession with the subject. On highway billboards, in magazine ads, in bestselling novels, and in almost every form from high art to low language, sexual innuendo dominates.

In Jewish life, sexual intimacy is also a big issue, but in perhaps a more resolved sense than in contemporary society. Jewish intimacy contains the highest potential for spirituality, as a means through. How a married couple expresses their holiness. At its highest, the sexual union in a Jewish marriage brings holiness beyond the household, into the world at large. This happens through the spiritual, emotional, and physical bond of husband and wife.

According to Jewish thought, a husband and wife are originally one soul before birth, split in half when the first of the two is conceived. Marriage—and more specifically intimacy between husband and wife—represents the reunion of halves as a single entity.

In describing the reunion that marital relations represent, the Torah tells us, "Therefore shall a man leave his father and mother and cleave unto his wife, and they shall become one flesh" (Genesis 2:24).

Oneness, the central goal of Jewish marriage, is not easy to achieve. By marriageable age, each individual has a unique history and experience, not to mention distinct likes and dislikes.

Fortunately, Jewish marriage itself provides tools for reconciling the divergent backgrounds of husband and wife, without promoting loss of individual identity. One such tool is the practice of family purity, with the mikvah (ritual bath) as its centerpiece. Historically, the mikvah has played a critical role in Jewish life, so much so that the rabbis of the Talmud ruled that a community without both a mikvah and a synagogue must first build a mikvah. While mikvah and family purity were once part and parcel of Jewish life, to this day, their practice provides stability and richness for a significant percentage of observant Jews.

The word "mikvah" means "collection." A mikvah is a pool that collects natural water from rain, a river, or an underground spring untouched by human hands. Though a mikvah looks something like a small pool or bath, it is truly a spiritual tool, rather than an entity connected to personal hygiene. In fact, a user must be perfectly physically clean before immersion.

Jewish men and women alike immerse in the mikveh before engaging in certain ritual acts. In the practice of family purity, the woman immerses following a period of physical separation from her husband that commences with the onset of menstruation. On the eve of the night the couple is to resume relations, the wife enters the waters of the mikvah, where she says a prayer inviting God to sanctify her forthcoming intimacy with her husband. Her immersion marks the start of renewed physical intimacy between husband and wife. This phase of their relationship lasts until the start of her next period.

The significance of the mikvah in this monthly change of status in a marriage can be understood by examining the spiritual potential of water itself. According to the Torah, water filled the world in the first stage of Creation. Genesis 1:2 reads, "...when the earth was astonishingly empty, with darkness upon the surface of the deep, and the Divine Presence hovered upon the surface of the waters..."

In connection with the primordial character of water, the waters of a mikveh at their time of collection remain untouched by humans. Hands (Jewish law mandates they come from rainfall or from an underground source). The waters of the mikveh have the potential to renew, refresh, and confer a sense of new beginning, reminiscent of the world at its very birth.

When a woman visits the mikvah, she, in a sense, emerges from the water and starts fresh, unencumbered by past obstacles to her personal growth and vision. After visiting the mikveh, she returns home to imbue her marriage, family, and relationships with the cohesiveness and harmony that belong to every Jewish woman.

https://torah.org/learning/womenclass3/

25) Exercise (Physical Body) Recovery

Your journey to your goals will not be easy. Remember, it is just as important to recover as you take strides from now on. There's nothing wrong with taking a step back if it means you are still two steps ahead of where you started.

We will introduce many options so you can choose what is best for you. Many people do not have the luxury to use such items, but there are more convenient choices. There are exercises for our physical bodies, but there are also those for the mind and spirit. In this book, We will talk about the second kind.

Recovery is based on how much energy you have spent and the soreness you have suffered. You can choose whatever works for you and continue according to your level. Whether weekend warriors or professional athletes, we all need to allow our bodies to rest and recover after exercise, of course, depending on the level of mileage and work.

Recovery Methods

After your favorite exercise of choice, or even on days your body is aching, here are some proven recovery methods for you to consider.

Recovery option one:

1. Hydrotherapy (used by pro athletes): Salt bath or pine bark with 98-degree water for 15-20 minutes. A dip in the ocean is also a great option.

2. Cold method (suitable for all levels): Bathe with ice bags or take a cold bath for 15-20 minutes, preferably after a workout or game.

Recoveries option two:

1 Jacuzzi (hot method): Try to do so once a week, an hour after your last workout of the week. For example, if you take Saturday off, do this on Fridays.

2. Acupuncture: It is best 23 hours after a workout to increase energy.

Out twice in one day, it is recommended to have a 10–15 minute massage right after the first and then 4 to 5 hours of rest between workouts.

But remember, Rambam says even 20 minutes a day is enough for the body; we don't need to go crazy, but I included all options to his level. For more details or to build your program, contact info@soulfit.com.

Active Recovery

Easy runs, foam rolling, stretching, hiking, and light outdoor activities. Our #1 Goal for the Soulfit Training Program:

Our theme quote for the program is "Get your body strong and your mind focused so you can better serve your soul!" —Soulfit

SECTION II

THE MIND

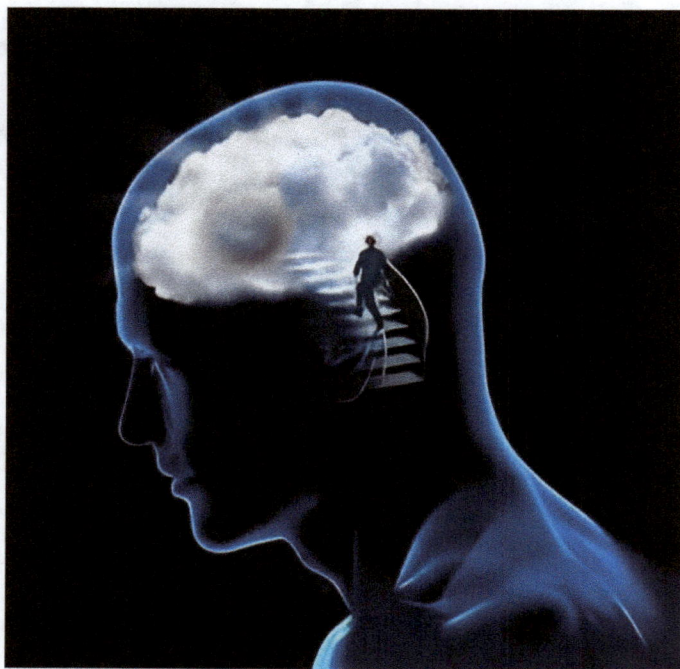

1) Habit

One of the most powerful forces of human nature is habit. Thus, for instance, a person might choose harmful foods to which he is accustomed over good food to which he is not accustomed.

So, how do we deal with cravings or bad habits that creep back into our minds? Whether you are a smoker who continues despite the risk of cancer or amputated limbs, or you crave bad foods before going to sleep, where does this urge come from? We must first accept that all humans have an animalistic pull toward immediate satisfaction. The animal's mind or soul does not weigh the consequences of its actions.

Positive behavior characteristics are not gained by doing positive acts but through the repetition of many positive acts. For example, giving a thousand gold coins to one charity will not accustom a person to traits of generosity, whereas giving one gold coin to a thousand different charities will. By repeating an act many times, an established behavioral or emotional pattern is formed. In contrast, one noble act represents arousal to good, after which that motivation may disappear. Rambam is teaching us a fundamental principle in human nature. Even a simple habit can affect our personal development more than a one-time significant motivational arousal.

The key is repetition.

In the early 1800s, eminent authorities explained how habits are formed. Learning a new language is a good example. A student learning how to pronounce words needs to know the letters of the alphabet. Then, the student learns how to join the letters together to form words. They must work extremely hard to learn this skill. Eventually, through much practice and repetition, this skill becomes ingrained.

Ultimately, it is a subconscious function, so the student has learned to read with ease and without conscious effort. We can apply this same process to the world of emotion. There are both conscious and subconscious factors in habit formation. No matter how small, even if it is forgotten immediately by the conscious mind, every feeling always leaves some impression on the memory.

Suppose one experiences this feeling a second time. In that case, it strengthens itself further with the first impression. Every time this feeling is experienced again, all the accumulated traces of the previous impressions combine from here. We can understand how the power of habit strengthens even the weakest feeling and how it creates learned desires, which intensify. Thus, over time, the most insignificant string of experiences can accumulate to become strong enough to overwhelm even superior experiences.

2) How to Let Go of Bad Habits and Learn Good Ones

Shift Our Perception

Once we first intellectually understand these points, it will help our willpower to overcome bad habits.

Subconscious Accumulation Process

Once we repeat and continue to learn and act on these mechanics, they will become habitual. Little by little, every experience, feeling, and image takes on a new meaning. This internal process affects every aspect of our personality and behavior.

Change Begins

These new experiences soon become new habits over time, and we can see that change begins and ends with perception. Thus, it starts with a shift in perception and ultimately ends with a behavior change. Yet, it is only through habit that we can internalize any new In perception and a behavior change.

These were summarized from The Path of the Just (chapter 23) by Moshe Chaim Luzzatto.

Newly accumulated motivations can overcome even the most entrenched habits, addictions, and cravings. Be patient. These things can take years to master. But if you keep learning and working at it, you will become a master regarding your choices, which will bring you great joy.

3) Focus

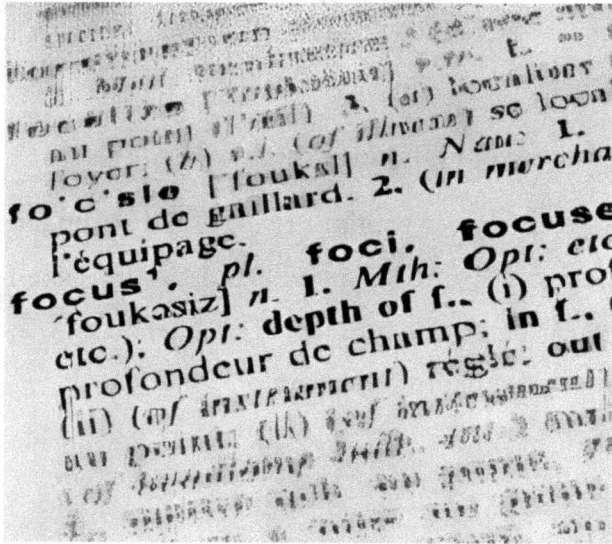

To have control of our minds, we must have focus. A focused An individual has a clear-cut direction and purpose in life. Rabbi Judah the Prince (Yehuda Ha Nasi, or, simply, Rebbe) would say, "Which is the right path for a man to choose for himself?
Whatever is harmonious for the one who does it and harmonious for humankind."

Here is a series of questions that will help you determine how focused you are as an individual:

- Who are you?
- What do you do? What drives you?
- What are you known for?

It is human nature to strive to be part of some community. This drive will usually begin early in childhood when we become influenced by others. We all want to identify with something. Maybe you are drawn to writing, the theater, or the worlds of athletics, academics, or music.

Notice the word choice in that last sentence: "Maybe you are drawn to..." And not, "Maybe you are talented at drawing or music..." Not everyone can be great at everything. If you try to do too many things, you will be mediocre at all, like most people. Mediocrity is not the way to be your best or to become a legend. Fame and wealth will not come overnight, but fulfillment should be your primary focus.

It is okay to have hobbies and enjoy other things you are interested in, but you must focus if you want to be great at something. So, focus In the one area that you identify with most.

Commitment is important. People are afraid to commit to jobs, hobbies, and even the person they love because we change daily and do the things we like. Sometimes, we are not even sure of things to begin with. However, it makes little sense to worry about the future.

Instead, dedicate your talents and energies to what you are passionate about now. That is a big part of happiness. If you find joy or contentment in what you are doing, you can indeed achieve success. Yes, many times, we must do things we do not like. But mostly, we should do something that facilitates who and what we are as individuals.

To be a world-class athlete or musician, it takes about ten thousand hours of focused practice. So, at an average of four hours every day, five days a week, this would mean somewhere in the real neighborhood of ten years of concentrated effort to become exceptional. But, of course, this does not mean that you will be the best; it just means that you will have paid your dues to compete at the highest levels.

Think about that for a while. World-class musicians, professional athletes, elite spiritual rabbis, and actors you see on your TV spent thousands of hours practicing, learning, and failing before they ever earned any substantial money or fame. But, of course, there are a few exceptions.

You will always find people who have become famous because of wealthy parents, great connections, or just "luck." However, the skill cannot be faked in many fields, such as science, music, and sports.

How have you invested ten thousand hours of your time? Into what are you prepared to invest ten thousand hours? If you are doing it solely for the money, it will not happen. You cannot put that much effort into something just for a future paycheck.

You need to sustain the drive and excitement when you are doing tedious repetitions of daily practice. Practicing music scales for four hours and learning spirituality through swimming hundreds of laps in a pool is not always glamorous. Nevertheless, top-level people in every field do these things to achieve personal excellence and mastery in their chosen endeavors.

For most of us, choosing a focus is incredibly hard. We all want to do many things. I want to start a new business, write a book, travel the world, play in a rock band, and go back to school. I am as greedy as the next person; I want to have everything. We will not accomplish very much if we try to do everything while concentrating on none of our talents.

If you want to be world-class or excel in anything, you need to channel your focus on the God-given gift that defines you. Here are some critical reasons why focus is vital: You will improve at one thing faster than if you try to master many things. Concentrating on that gift or talent minimizes distractions, tours, and diversions. You will always think about better ways, new ideas, and opportunities to share your gift with the world with only one goal. As a result, the quantity and quality of your efforts will increase tremendously. Singular, concentrated effort changes your identity. You become known as the person who does that one thing. Concentrating on one thing, in particular, is vital because you will start gaining support, help, and encouragement from friends and acquaintances.

Your confidence and determination will increase with additional support, and you will probably get significant help in your effort. Once you become known as the person doing your one thing, you will be introduced to people who can help you. You will meet like-minded people with whom you can share ideas. You may even find new investors or partners.

Once you become known as the person doing your one thing, you will be introduced to people who can help you. You will meet like-minded people with whom you can share ideas. You may even find new investors or partners.

Multitaskers rarely achieve world-class success. Multitasking is just another excuse for procrastination.

Success comes from focus:

- Focus on GOD.
- Focus on yourself.
- Focus on family.
- Focus on friends.
- Focus on your passion, and finally,
- Focus on leaving the world a better place than you found it.

Developing and sustaining focus is quite difficult for many people, so we recommend this order of priorities to work on focus. First and foremost, we are not at the level to advise others unless we know their situation. We will share what Rambam says about prioritizing and then give some humble tips:

In his commentary on the Mishnah, Avot 1:14, Rambam says to make your Torah study of primary importance and all your other affairs secondary. If they come your way, then it is a good thing, and if not, there is no loss in their absence. Similarly, in Hilchot De'ot 2:7, the Rambam quotes Avot 4:10, "Minimize your business involvement and occupy yourself with Torah."

A person need not fear that involvement in Torah study will prevent him from achieving prosperity. The Talmud, Berachot 35b, relates: The previous generations' sages made their study primary and business affairs secondary and achieved notable success with both.

Do not say, "I will study when I have free time," for perhaps you will never have free time.

1. Focus on the one GOD who created this world and what He wants from you for your well-being.
2. Focus on your career/job: Pick the activity that defines you and helps you be the best version of yourself.
3. Focus on your marriage: Choose that one eternal partner. Then, if it did not work the first time, get back on the horse and try again. It will come. GOD wants you to be with your soul's other half.
4. Focus on your children (if applicable): With GOD's blessing, you bring children into the world, teach and raise them to Torah and good deeds, and raise them where you may have fallen.
5. Focus on your parents/family of origin: Never forget who brought you into the world. Appreciation and respect are essential.
6. Focus on friends/community: If you have free time after your 95, please give and help the people around you with kindness and charity.
7. Focus on Eretz Yisrael: It is crucial to have time left in your week or month to keep learning more about Eretz Yisrael and how important it is to help protect and support this sacred land, the center of the world's spirituality.

8. Focus on the World: Share anything you feel you have learned from this book with others. If we all learn to share positive thoughts, we may fix our broken world.

Sages say that in the future, the entire world will be on the level of Eretz Yisrael, and all of Eretz Yisrael will be at the level of Yerushalayim!

4) The Power of Joy

No matter what comes our way, we must constantly remind ourselves that it is for our very best. Any challenge is an opportunity to grow. Just like a loving father loves his kids and must discipline them from time to time for their benefit, GOD may need to do so with us. So many times, curveballs are thrown at us to get our attention.

The more we view our relationship with God as a loving father, the further we can go. Joy gives us the strength to go further and further on our physical and spiritual paths. When man harnesses his biological urges as instructed by GOD, life becomes a beautiful process. Once you have practiced and made this routine, you can take it to the next level by deepening your love with another.

For instance, the union of husband and wife becomes a sublime expression of their love for each other, a love deepened by their mutual love of GOD. All vitality of their souls is given over to the work of creation and building, fulfilling the commandments of GOD.

Excerpts from Rabbi Nachman's Tikkun (compiled and translated by Avraham Greenbaum).

5) Charity: Elevating the Material

Giving to others strengthens our minds. The merit of giving charity, or tzedakah, has the power to protect us from harm and prolong our lives. In the unforgettable words of Maimonides, "A person puts his life and energy into earning a living. The money he gives away contains his very life." Thus, giving charity is a way of uplifting all his sins. "When a person gives part of his income to charity, he elevates all his material affairs. Therefore, charity is the choice part of what he earns. In giving it away, he shows that his primary goal in earning money is for spiritual ends. You help yourself first and then others around you with this mindset; all material affairs are thus drawn in this direction."

There are eight levels of charity. Maimonides wrote about them, and you can read about them in greater detail in his book, Mishneh Torah (Laws of Charity, 10:714).

6) Ways to Respond to Anger

Realize you are not in control.

Our sages refer to anger as idolatry (Maimonides—Laws of Behavior 2:2). When you think you are the master of the universe and things inexplicably do not bend to your will, you explode. You are not GOD. Be humble and realize you are not in control.

Give yourself a timeout.

When we are angry, we are not rational. We say things we do not mean to say. We can do terrible things that we usually would never consider doing. That is why the Talmud tells us not to discipline our kids when angry; we are not objective, and at that moment, any action is not for the child's sake (Talmud—Moed Katan 17a). So, remove yourself from the situation, count to 10, breathe deeply, cool off, and get a grip. It is not okay to go to bed angry. Keeping your anger bottled up creates stress and internal pressure that is bound to erupt negatively. You can get it off your chest by writing an uncensored letter to the person you are feeling angry toward; express how you feel, and do not hold back. Then rip up the letter. The letter is for your eyes only.

Use anger as your teacher.

What is making you angry? What does it trigger inside of you? What message are you taking from this hurt? Anger is often a result of more deeply seated frustrations and is based on a distorted view of the situation. Figure out what is triggering your anger and objectively evaluate if you are reading the situation right. There is a great book we highly advise reading on anger by Rabbi Zelig Pliskin. He is a noted psychologist and prolific author of 24 books.

Forgive.

Forgiveness does not mean condoning or justifying any misdeeds. Instead, it means seeing the person who hurt you as an injured person. It is giving up your desire for revenge. It is untying the knots that keep you emotionally entwined and prevent you from healing.

Everything GOD does is for good.

One of Rabbi Akiva's maxims is "All that the Merciful One does, He does for good" (Talmud—Berachot 60b). Everything GOD does is out of love. It is for our good. We may not see the big picture right now, especially amid anger, but stop and ask yourself, "Why do you? I need this right now. How is this for my ultimate good?" The answer may surprise you.

7) The Letter

In the 13th century, the Jewish people found a grand champion who pleaded their cause and defended their faith against a cruel attack. This grand champion was Rabbi Moses ben Nachman Gerondi, known as Ramban or Nachmanides. He was called Gerondi after his native town, Gerona, Spain, where he was born in 1195. He was born into a noble family, which included many prominent Talmudists.

At 72, the Ramban left his beloved community, his famous Yeshivah, friends, and native land. Instead, he set out for the Land of Israel, hoping to find peace and solace there.

Unfortunately, he found the Holy Land in great desolation; the Jewish communities were scarce and scattered; young and old alike were poor and ignorant of Jewish knowledge. So, the Ramban at once began a campaign to improve the position of his brethren in the Holy Land, both spiritually and materially. He reorganized the communities, set up schools, rebuilt the synagogues, and gave public lectures and discourses. Here is when he wrote his famous commentary on the Torah and other works. Moreover, he sent copies to his native land and sent the Zohar from Israel to Spain. They're the first to introduce that holy book to the West.

Ramban died at 7. He wrote a letter in his later years to his son. This letter was sent to his son in Catalonia regarding the act of humility and controlling one's anger.

He instructed him to read this once every week, teach it to others, and learn it by heart to train them in their youth to fear heaven. The Ramban assured him that his wishes would be fulfilled from heaven on the day that he reads this letter, and whoever will accustom themselves to saying it will spare themselves from all pains. They are assured of inheriting the world to come (from the book Me'ulephet Sappirim).

A person who can control their anger is genuinely great, as our Rabbis teach us, "Who is a hero? One who controls his destructive urges" (Ethics of Our Fathers 4:1). A person who can show self-control will find that this is the key to success at work and at home. To see the complete letter translated in Hebrew with an English translation, see

8) Anger and Income

The Hebrew word for "anger" is Kaas. The root of this word comes from the Kisay Hakavod, or the Chair in Heaven. This Heavenly Chair is a spiritually powerful item. Sages say that our income (which in Hebrew is parnassa, which refers to something sent down to us from Heaven) is determined.

Thus, the Jewish sages revealed that a big factor controlling our income is handling our anger. In two types of situations, one is with ourselves, and the other is with the person closest to us, which in most cases is our spouse (for married couples). Thus, Kaas in Hebrew is associated not only with the word kise ("chair") but also with Keter ("crown").

Men: Treat the woman you have chosen as the crown on your head. Treat her like royalty, utterly devoid of anger, and you will be shocked at the results. Women are men's mirrors; however the men behave, the women respond. Therefore, you get what you give.

It is the man's responsibility to set the tone. In short, treat your wife as your crown (Keter), and then you will be the king. Learn to control your anger with yourself and others, and God will send down His blessing from His Kise Hakavod. (His Chair of spiritual royalty.)

9) Power of Speech

In the Jewish tradition, our holy sages teach us that GOD created the universe through words, and He sustains it continuously through the power of speech. Thus, our sages clarify that our words genuinely uphold the world. "The world was created through ten utterances" (Ethics of the Fathers 5:1 Pirkei Avot). There are four elements used by the Creator: fire, water, wind, and earth.

Earth is the lowest element, representing action, but it cannot take action unless the first three activate it. Like all other creatures, humans can be described as made up entirely of these four essential elements. Our sages say that speaking activates the elements, enabling them to be helpful in the world. For example, when a person opens their mouth to say something, the physical breath they exhale to express the words is warm. Speech is related to the element of fire. In the mouth, the moisture from the saliva is water. The exhaling as they pronounce the words is wind. These three elements make up a person's speech, which leads to the attribute of action, or what we bring to this world, the earth. Speech exhibits so much power, and great care must be taken when we speak to make sure that we are correctly harnessing the forces of the universe.

Every word that we utter has a profound impact on our lives and those around us. Offensive or angry words can have seriously damaging, far-reaching effects on both us and the world. Therefore, choose to use positive, encouraging words to help you and your loved ones.

Feel honored and blessed when someone, anyone, blesses you with positive words. You should answer, "Amen," with enthusiasm, as this can change the course of your direction on this precious journey.

10) The Power of Thought

When a person thinks of evil or negative thoughts, they are continuously afflicted by their feelings. The mere thoughts of depression, anger, jealousy, hatred, etc., can have detrimental effects. Even when they are mere thoughts, they lead to even greater trouble for the soul, with no action being carried out.

For instance, the Hebrew word for happiness (simcha) is the same as (thoughts) machshava. Thinking good will be good. Also, another secret about thoughts and the word for pressure (lachatz): if you add the letter "hey," you have hatzlacha. Hey also represents Hashem, so when we add Hashem to your pressure, we get success.

Sages tell us that our soul is actually in our minds. This means that our thoughts occupy a very lofty place in the supernatural, spiritual worlds. Thinking is a spiritual endeavor, which is why it corresponds to a higher and more religious world than speech or action does, both of which are more physical than thought. So how can I govern my thoughts and direct them to more valuable channels?

By the power of speech.

When people are careful about what they say, they achieve this by thinking about what they want to say before saying it. In this way, they are controlling not only their speech but also their thoughts.

When we think about our speech and respect its ability to have more positive thoughts, we can head towards a better direction in our lives.

Power to Think and Act. When we think positive thoughts, they will help us carry out positive actions as well.

A person's negative thoughts will remind them of bad times; positive thoughts will remind them of good times. Dwelling on unfortunate events will lead to depression and weaken us, slowing our growth and success.

Suggestions on how to think and act positively: Whenever a negative thought comes to mind, we must begin the habit and practice by replacing it with positive thinking: "I will make it, I will succeed, I will be great, etc." It will take time to train your brain, but soon, this will become a habit.

Once a person experiences a positive mind, they rely more on God and less on themselves. You rely less on your mental capabilities and more on GOD's mercy and kindness.

I have listed spiritual tools that GOD has passed down through the sages to help us. You cannot rely on sages, humankind, this book, or me solely. You can only use this book as a tool, bearing in mind that our hope, trust, and reliability must come from GOD, for humankind makes mistakes, and only GOD is perfect and divine.

11) Power of Imagination

Imagination is a spiritual power that GOD grants as a gift for us to use in positive ways. Many people often have negative thoughts, whether from painful or frightening experiences growing up or current events.

Such negative thoughts include fear, anger, worry, despair, and other draining feelings. We will give you the tools to understand and overcome these negatively influenced emotions.

As we mentioned above, GOD instilled in us both an animal instinct and a pure instinct. Both are good and are used for different reasons. They both put different things in our imagination, and soon, you will realize them both and understand how to decipher one from the other. Then, you will use each in the right way and 58   for   the right reasons, as we need both. For example, we need animal energy to rise in the morning, the strength to work, and to fight for good causes.

We need divine energy to give people the benefit of the doubt and help us learn godly wisdom to apply to understanding, care, and love, all in many situations. One of the primary purposes of our imagination is to help us understand the existence of goodness in the world. It is also used to realize GOD's existence and arrive at a complete understanding of the Garden of Eden (Gan Eden in Hebrew); we should now actually have an image of that ancient garden in our mind's eye.

Tools to combat negative imaginations:

1. Shift Perception.

2. Subconscious Accumulation Process.

3. When perception changes, change begins.

We can fight back against negative imagination by filling our minds with positive, joyful, and loving thoughts. Put away thoughts of despair and anguish. This will become a habit in time, and you will see an improved you in all aspects of your life: work, relationships, dreams, aspirations, etc.

The power of imagination can indeed influence our emotions, and the more we work on the actual construction of our minds, the more joyful we will become. The tools above will ultimately increase our faith and trust in GOD, for which he will repay us in due time with his abundant kindness, or Chesed (including His mercy).

12) Power of Free Will

The Creator gave us the ability to choose freely, and therefore, we can decide to think positive or negative thoughts. As long as the change is desired in a person's situation, we must have positive thoughts. Those thoughts, together with trust in Hashem, can change our lives for the better.

You can control your thoughts by using free will to focus on those things you choose to think about. Remember this: no one can think of a positive and a negative thought at the same time. So, if we decide to think positively and practice it, unwanted thoughts will disappear automatically.

We cannot change the past, but we can affect and influence the future. When we understand that we have the free will to choose our thoughts and let our imaginations go, we can become masters of our emotions. If we focus on praying and thinking about beautiful things, these are the outcomes we will get. In conclusion, our thoughts determine a great deal of how our lives will play out.

13) The Third Eye and the Quarter Pounder

This next section may shock many, but it is vital to building awareness to live a more holistic, organic, and natural life. The third eye is a gland in the brain affected by substances we take into our bodies and what we are exposed to. In medical terms, it is called the pineal gland.

Why is this important?

The pineal gland is perhaps the most spiritually sensitive part of the brain. Many sages say we can build up our bodies, minds, and

Souls are to reach a level of divine inspiration, which is called the Ruach HaKodesh in Hebrew. Now, many have never reached this level during their whole lives, but some can. Sometimes it is gifted to people; sometimes it is earned.

The famed Baba Sali, or Rabbi Israel Abuhatzeira, was a leading Moroccan Sephardic rabbi and a Kabbalist renowned for his ability to work miracles through his prayers. His burial place in Netivot, Israel, has become a shrine for prayers and petitioners. He could perform many miracles by accessing the Ruach HaKodesh and helping people with life-threatening situations. There are countless stories of his purity and loving kindness. We are not claiming that this book or a special diet will help you reach his level of piety, but we can suggest a starting point or shed some light on bringing spirituality back into our lives. We will start by examining what forces in the world are damaging or blocking the light.

First step: If you want to develop this gland and become conscious of it during meditation, you must understand what helps and hurts it.

America has, unfortunately, become the world's leader in obesity and fast-food chains. As a result, many foods we consume are very harmful to our bodies (especially our gut and the pineal gland). The more junk food and preserved food we eat, the more we damage this gland, which we feel can be part of our spiritual focus. Even an urban legend asserts that there is a slightly sinister plan among various elite groups to dumb down the unsuspecting masses by adulterating the food supply with additives, flavorings, and other artificial substances.

Ingredients.

We will discuss the importance of "gut health" from Dr. Helfgott's article: Most of us have heard the term "gut health" and know that keeping it in good standing is desirable and advantageous to our overall well-being. But what does it truly mean to have a healthy gut? Michele Helfgott, MD, PPG–Integrative Medicine, helps answer this question while discussing the importance of a balanced gut microbiome and the steps we can take to improve it.

What is gut health?

Believe it or not, your gut microbiome is the foundation of your health. Good gut health occurs when you have a balance between the good (helpful) and bad (potentially harmful) bacteria and yeast in your digestive system. 80% of your immune system is in the gut, and the majority of your body's serotonin is, too. This means if your gut isn't healthy, then your immune system and hormones won't function, and you will get sick.

Why is gut health so important for our overall health and well-being?

As previously mentioned, your gut is the foundation of everything. It aids in the digestion of the foods you eat, absorbs nutrients, and uses them to fuel and maintain your body. So, if your gut is imbalanced and your immune system isn't working properly, serotonin and hormones won't either, making it more challenging to stay healthy.

Your gut is also where your body gets rid of metabolic waste and toxins. However, if you have an unhealthy gut, your body will struggle to rid itself of those toxins. If this occurs, it can cause many issues, including chronic fatigue, chronic illnesses, and inflammation throughout the body. That's why people experience symptoms such as brain fog, diarrhea, constipation, gas, joint pain, etc. You may not realize it, but the brain is the second gut; therefore, if your gut isn't working, your brain is struggling too.

What factors affect the health of our gut?

While several factors can contribute to poor gut health, some of the most common can include:

- **Stress:** This increases intestinal permeability (leaky gut), tipping the scales toward an imbalance of more bad than good bacteria in the gut.

- **Poor nutrition:** Most people eat processed food and sugar, which can harm the beneficial bacteria in your gut and contribute to or cause inflammation throughout the body.

- **Long-term use of antibiotics and antacids**: They all decrease B12 within the gut, which is essential for cell production, brain function, and energy. They also kill the good bacteria that live in

Your gut. However, it's important to note that there is a time and a place for these medications, but it's best to consult with your physician before using them.

What are the signs of an unhealthy gut?

An unhealthy gut can appear as gas, bloating, constipation, and diarrhea, but it can present itself in many other forms as well. Autoimmune disorders like Hashimoto's disease, rheumatoid arthritis, Type 1 diabetes, and multiple sclerosis (MS), where your immune system is attacking different parts of the body, can also be a sign of an unhealthy gut. Brain fog, headaches, poor concentration and memory, fatigue, chronic pain, trouble sleeping, and issues with cravings or bad moods are also symptoms and critical indicators of a poor microbiome.

What steps can someone take to get a healthy gut or improve it?

Fortunately, many patients find they can balance their microbiome and heal their gut by managing their stress levels, practicing mindfulness, eating healthy, getting enough hours of sleep a night, and exercising.

However, a subset of patients may need more than just those things, but it's essential to start with those items first. Once you build a foundation, you can get fancier with pre, pro, and post biotics.

Integrative Chiropractic care can also help? It's a system of focusing on the underlying causes of your condition, not limited to your spine only. One recommendation is Barry Lieberman, DC, ACN; he is trying to make America healthy again, one individual at a time. https://wholebodycures.com/

Final thoughts

Remember, healing your gut will take time, dedication, and consistency. Your microbiome didn't get unhealthy overnight, so you aren't going to fix it overnight either. Eating healthy and managing your stress will go a long way in getting you on the road to recovery and optimal gut health.

We highly suggest finding physicians or health practitioners who are God fearing and really care for your own well-being. One powerful spiritual tip is that Tzadikim have advised that when eating food with right kavana (intentions/meditations) that this food can help heal us. Rabbi Eliyahi Netaneli Shalita has advised me that GOD has created nature to have all the healing elements; if one can heal his body with good food; minerals, and vitamins, that is best; of course, if one is in an emergency state, he must seek medical care (it's a mitzvah) and advice to do everything he needs to stay alive.

Antibiotics; even some steroid medication; can help save your life, so if you need you take them. I personally had experience with asthma and pneumonia, and had to take strong medicine. It was not fun, but

In case of an emergency, we must do everything to stay alive. There are many ways to prevent things, and we must do our best. The challenge is that today's Western Medicine is not always in line with Rambam's view of healing the body as a whole (one unit, not separately. Western and Eastern medicine refer to two different systems of medicine. Western medicine prescribes specific drugs for a disease. In contrast, naturopathic medicine focuses on treating the person as a whole rather than just their symptoms.

Some physicians have combined Western, natural, and Eastern practices. You should pray to find a good doctor who treats your body as a whole. For instance, he should advise eating healthy, exercising, and finding ways to lower stress. If not, you must help yourself. Get stronger in all ways you can. We must pray for this; also, try to put your faith in God and allow your body to help heal itself.

Hashem miraculously made the body and allowed it to be healed. Take excellent care to strengthen your gut and immune system. You will be better able to fight off medical issues. Now this also means your body, your spirit, your soul, and your environment!! Yes, that means good water, air, food, love!!! And positive thinking. We will move to another emerging topic about technology awareness.

Cell phones and computers are becoming the norm for many of our children, and this movement is quite dangerous. It may be too early to see damage from the new 5G networks, but that does not mean we should not build awareness of the subject for our safety.

Instead, we should let the experts share their research and insights. Martin Pall, Professor Emeritus of Biochemistry, Washington State University, summarized the 5G potential health threats: Increased risk of blindness from the four major causes of blindness: cataracts, macular degeneration, glaucoma, and retinal detachment.

- Risk of tinnitus, hearing loss, and deafness.
- Increased risk of male infertility and widespread reductions in sperm count.
- Increased risk of melanoma, leukemia, and possibly other types of cancer, particularly in children.
- Potential impact on the peripheral nervous system, leading to near-universal neuropathic pain and peripheral neuropathy.
- Risk of thyroid dysfunction because of the location of the thyroid gland near the surface of the body.
- Impact on immune system cells, possibly leading to autoimmune diseases and immunodeficiency.
- Impact on erythrocytes leading to stacking of the erythrocytes into rouleaux (long chains) and also erythrocyte lysis, leading to lower tissue oxygenation.
- Ecosystem disruption affects insects (including bees and other pollinators), birds, small mammals, and many forms of plant life.

"Mechanisms by which health effects are exerted have been shown to include oxidative stress, damage to mitochondria, damage to cell membranes, and via these mechanisms, an impaired blood brain barrier, constriction of blood vessels and impaired blood flow to the brain, and triggering of autoimmune reactions," Beatrice Golomb, MD, Ph.D., a lead professor at the University of California, San Diego (UCSD).

She contends that the broad deployment of 5G will expose Americans to far more continuous EMF, potentially causing more significant oxidative stress and all the physiological changes that go along with it.

"Following a large exposure that depresses antioxidant defenses, magnifying vulnerability to future exposures, some people no longer tolerate many other forms and intensities of electromagnetic radiation that previously caused them no problem, but this group deserves the right to avoid these exposures," wrote Golumb.

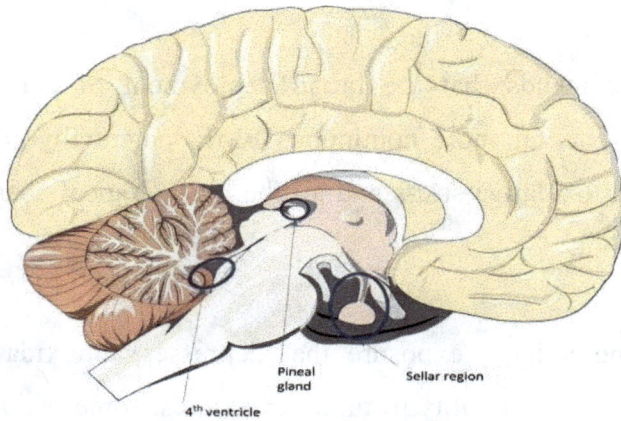

Pineal gland   Sellar region

4th ventricle

"Each new rollout of electromagnetic technology for which exposure is obligatory swells the ranks of those who develop problems with electromagnetic fields (EMF)," she argues. "As each new technology leading to further exposure to electromagnetic radiation is introduced—and particularly introduced in a fashion that prevents vulnerable individuals from avoiding it, a new group becomes sensitized to [its] health effects."

Golumb has assessed hundreds of patients suffering from symptoms that she believes are associated with RF exposure: headaches, ringing ears, insomnia, and longer-lasting chronic conditions, including cancer, infertility, and neurological damage. She and Dr. Pall are not alone in their concerns.

Over 180 scientists and doctors from 35 countries sent an appeal to the United Nations and World Health Organization leaders, asserting.

Those agencies responsible for "setting safety standards have failed to impose sufficient guidelines to protect the public" from hazardous EMF.

Constant use of wireless technology may also have a secondary and indirect negative effect on cognition. Mobile devices encourage us to outsource our memories to computers. For example, our cell phones keep our calendars and remind us of important events. Texting, with spell check, has replaced writing, and many people no longer exercise the forms of memory associated with spelling and grammar.

Tools like "smart refrigerators" can be programmed to sense the food and beverage products they contain, notifying users when their favorite foods are running low and, sometimes, automatically ordering more.
According to German neuroscientist Manfred Spitzer, this promotes the underuse and deterioration of short-term memory pathways, a condition he calls "digital dementia."

Rees agrees: "Our dependence on technology is dumbing us down. With your brain, you use it, or you lose it. We need to remember things and take responsibility for our actions. So many of us are already deeply immersed in a culture of technology that is unnecessary and is making us less competent as people, needing it more."
The notion that technology is addictive is not metaphorical. "Devices are like a stimulant. They are dopaminergic," says Rees, citing the work of addiction psychologist Nicholas Kardaras, author of Glow Kids. Kardaras contends that the constant glow of device screens can be as dopamine-activating to young brains as ill-suited images and

videos.

According to the AAP, "Problems begin when media use displaces physical activity, hands-on exploration, face-to-face social interaction in the real world, which is critical to learning." Device dependence is not just child's play, though. Health experts warn young and old tech users alike about the dangers of technology addiction, and, around the world, "tech wellness" is becoming big business.

Methods for treating it have been explored. There are even groups specializing in the treatment of teenage tech addiction, including digital detox summer camps for children and behavioral health programs for video game-addled kids.

14)Minimizing RF Risk

Not everyone can afford a digital detox on the beach, but there are steps we can all take to minimize our exposure to RF radiation.

A few good starting points are reducing screen time, particularly at night, before bed, and unplugging or turning devices on airplane mode when they are not in use. In addition, Rees tells cell phone users to avoid holding devices directly against their heads. Instead, use the phone's speaker function with the device set down on a table. She also encourages clinicians to educate themselves and their patients about personal and community-wide risks of RF exposure. The nonprofit group Physicians for Safe Technology teaches health professionals about the potential adverse effects of technology and provides tools for diagnosing and treating sensitive patients.

What's Going On? | Dr. Dietrich Klinghardt Dr. Dietrich Klinghardt says, "You know that towards the end of last century, at the beginning of the century, there will be movement driven by big corporations to take the soul away from people to disconnect people from the higher world and to do that we have to destroy the pineal gland in people we followed the research on that and amazingly what we found the pineal gland is the most sensitive part of our central nervous system and it is highly sensitive to four things: aluminum, glyphosate, fluoride, and WiFi. We are the only country in the world that has pushed these four things on everybody in the last sixty years.

Well, folks, there is plenty of interesting information, and later on, we will speak more about the danger of the internet (without a good filter).

We advise those who can, do power down when you are not using the device, use the speaker or headset, and perhaps try to take a break from the city and go to GOD's beautiful natural surroundings to do some deep breathing and meditate. Pray for the wellness of yourself, your loved ones, and the World. Meditation and prayer (Tefilot in Hebrew) might help activate healthy bioelectric energy! With practice, you can direct this energy to the pineal gland. You can stimulate and help it open up to be more aware of your spiritual surroundings. For your meditation to be effective, your mind must become still enough to merge the scattered energy in your body.

We advise you to focus on the Hebrew letters, as they have potent effects on cleansing. On a side note, turmeric and apple cider vinegar can also help cleanse the body and help the glands. Fasts help replenish the gland as well.

Look at the Jewish calendar for further information regarding fast dates. Be aware of the high amount of gluten used in today's baking business. Look for more ancient bread options, such as spelt or sourdough.

We will end with a prescription given to me by one of my health professionals: Prescription for Optimal Health. "Drink purified or spring water in glass containers throughout the day.

- Eat and drink smaller amounts more frequently.
- Take deeper abdominal breaths through your nose.
- Exercise regularly.
- Sweat.
- Sunshine without burning.
- Ground yourself through direct contact with earth, grass, or a tree (earthing) to help balance energy.
- Avoid processed foods, GMO foods, fried foods, trans fats, vegetable oils, high fructose products, corn syrups, and artificial ingredients.

sweeteners.

- Limit EMF exposure from WiFi, Bluetooth, alarm clocks, cell phones, computer equipment, etc. Health comes with proper Nourishment + Avoidance + Detoxification... "Charles W. Penick, M.D.

Diplomate, American Board of Family Medicine. We are quite proud of you for passing the Body and Mind section. For many, the most complex and challenging awaits—but keep striving forward. It will all be worth it.

SECTION III

THE SOUL

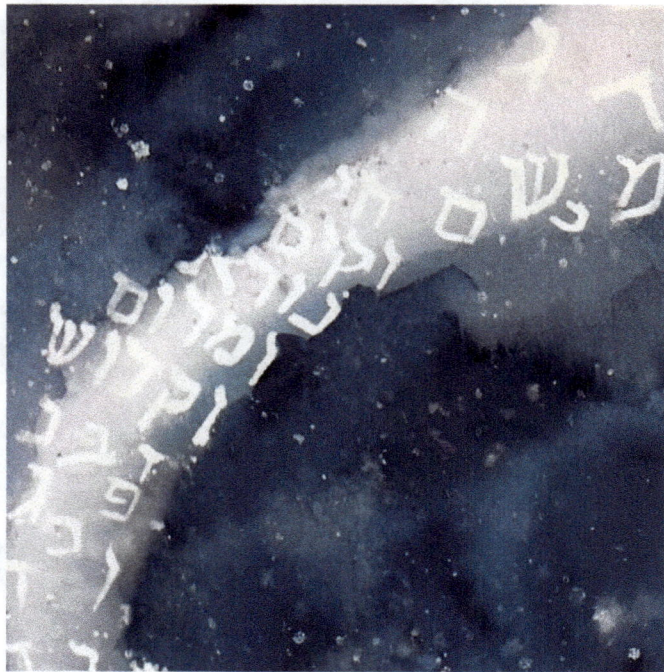

1)Our #1 Rule for Training

"Get your body strong and your mind focused so you can better serve your Soul!" Both your soul and body need care. You strengthen your body by respecting and treating it well. You strengthen your soul by training it through divine information, wisdom, ethics, and prayer. If we tend to the body alone, we neglect its purpose: serving the soul. If you focus on the soul alone, you neglect your body's needs.

Do not neglect your body's needs; do not overwork or weaken it because it will weaken your body and soul.

Just as we take care of our bodies and minds, we must also seek to care for our souls. The soul needs a healthy balance, just like the physical aspects of our existence, similar to how our bodies need the correct amount of protein, carbs, etc.

Our souls need the same stability and care. This process starts with understanding the truth that our soul came from a Master Creator. Just like a chair or a computer did not fall from the sky, they had a master designer or creator. It is only common sense that the more sophisticated the product, the more sophisticated the designer.

2)History of the Soul

"In the beginning, GOD created the heavens and the earth. Now the earth was astonishingly empty, and darkness was on the face of the deep, and the divine spirit of GOD was hovering over the face of the water, and GOD said, 'Let there be light,' and there was light..." 1
The Book of Genesis opens with the story of creation. GOD creates the world by speaking into the darkness/', T4 and calling into light, sky, land, vegetation, and living creatures for six days. Each day, He pronounces His works "good" (e.g., Genesis 1:4). He uses the Hebrew letters to put this all into being (more on this later).

Finally, on the sixth day, GOD declares His intention to make a being in His image, and He creates humankind to watch guard over planet Earth (Genesis 1:26). He fashions a human out of dust. We will try to condense this since there is so much information that an entire book can be written just on this. GOD saw that Man was alone and in need of a partner to populate the world, and so He formed a woman out of the man's rib.

GOD places the two people, Adam and Eve, in the idyllic Garden of Eden, encouraging them to procreate and enjoy the world fully; the only caveat is that he forbade them from eating from the Tree of the Knowledge of Good and Evil.
Life was perfect at this point. GOD lived through His Spirit here on Earth, and the world was perfect. So, what can we learn here?

GOD created the world with words, and those words are the Hebrew alphabet or, in Hebrew, the alphabet. Each letter is extraordinary and takes a unique role and a united role in creation. The Greeks gained the concept of an alphabet from a Semitic source, the ancient Phoenicians, influenced by the development of the Hebrew alphabet. (For a list of the letters of the alphabet and their pronunciations, see the appendix.)

Humans comprise everything from the earth: water, fire, air, and even the sky. GOD soon instructs Adam not to eat from one tree, His first commandment. Next, he decrees a challenge to test His creation with the wily snake or serpent, which GOD also created to exist in the Garden.

The snake comes along and entices Eve to eat from the forbidden tree (the tree of knowledge). This is an action that changes the course of history. However, with His infinite patience, kindness, and mercy, GOD gave Adam and Eve a chance to repent for not following the commandment not to eat from the tree. Some commentators say the Creator was going to destroy Eve, but He gave Adam a chance to repent first to avoid a harsher fate.

When he was alone, he asked Adam why he had disobeyed GOD's simple directive of avoiding the forbidden fruit. GOD asked Adam, "Where are you?" In essence, GOD was checking in on His newly created human to see Adam's reaction to having sinned. Unfortunately, instead of restoring

His integrity and repairing the damage his disobedience had caused, Adam took a more frightening route, thus incurring an even greater punishment. Adam should have taken responsibility for what he had done. But he pointed fingers at GOD and his wife instead of himself. Since Adam began blaming others for his crime, God expelled him from the Garden of Eden and distanced him from the close spirituality he once had.

From this, we have so much to learn about the role of husband and wife, taking responsibility, and what keeps GOD's divine spirit on this earth. We cannot list all the specific lessons and essential wisdom here, but we invite you to learn more by reading Genesis and the early sections of the Written Torah. Our History Continues.

The snake accomplished its mission, leaving humankind unable to live on this Earth with a pure and holy divine soul. This forced GOD to create another soul within man, called the animal soul (or evil inclination). This animalistic soul has a positive and negative side.
The positive side is the same as the originally pure soul we were created with. However, it takes a lot of practice to tell these two sides apart.

The Yetzer Hara (Hebrew for evil inclination/animal soul) is first represented to humankind as a diversion dressed up like a snake. However, we learn that the Yetzer Hara is meant to help us achieve growth in the trained mind and soul. Like how any challenge pushes us to see how we may react and how every great coach pushes us past what seems to be our limits, they expand what we can achieve.

Our free will gives us the capacity to achieve greatness.

We must control ourselves and never give in to our basic instincts. We must train our minds and bodies to filter and choose words and actions carefully and thoughtfully through the divine soul. It may sound harsh, but with time and training, it can be done.

Adam and Eve are expelled from the Garden of Eden. After that, they are then left to roam the Earth. GOD's punishment for the sin of the first humans was that Adam must work the land. Adam, who represents all humankind, is cursed to sweat from his brow to earn a living. He will have to work extra hard to grow and enjoy the food necessary for himself and his family's future.

Because of his direct and shameless disobedience of GOD's only prohibition, when he could have had his heart's desire and eaten from any other tree, Adam could no longer enjoy the once intimate and direct communion with his Creator, in a perfect, primeval Garden. Nor would life on this Earth as we know it ever again be as easy as before. Eve was placed in a natural state of clinging to or needing Adam and having pains during childbirth.

This state of affairs still exists today. Much of humanity is still required to sweat from its brow from hard work, while many women still experience pain during labor and childbirth. Any good news? Yes! Once we rectify ourselves and our sins, man will not have to sweat from his brow to earn a living, and women will no longer have pain in childbirth.

Even before the curse, the man needed the assistance of a woman to help him. She is essentially part of him (she was made from his rib. If he damages her, he hurts himself, and vice versa. In modern-day terms, it is a Win-Win or a Lose-Lose dynamic in the marriage arena. To reach the goal of uniting with GOD and the original divine spirit and soul, we must be united, men and women, to work together as a team. The story written above is but one approach; there are many facets and commentaries on creating the world from the Beresheet section of the Chumash.

Many schools of thought attribute sin to sinful speech, sexuality, and a simple sense of responsibility. Regardless of which school of thought you resonate with, it is important to appreciate them all.

This is the beauty of the Torah.

Next, when man was sent out of the Garden, his generation only grew stronger and waxed exceedingly in sin. Things got so bad that humankind forced GOD to destroy the world and start over. This occurred with the Great Flood.

It was around this time that a hero, Noah, emerged. He was the only man in his day who could conquer his anger, jealousy, lust, and desire for honor. He was fit to survive. We learn the precious and invaluable seven Noahide Laws from him, which must be taught and continuously preached to the world today.

3)Universal morality: the seven Noahide Laws

It is believed that the fundamental laws for all humanity were derived from Noah after the Flood. Noah is the parent of all humankind, hence the name Noahide (sometimes spelled Noachide) Laws. These seven laws, which all human beings need to follow if they want a true, genuine relationship with the Creator of the universe. Notice that there are not ten such laws, as in the famous Ten Commandments, primarily designed for the Jewish people.

These are the Seven Laws:

1) Do not murder.

2) Do not steal.

3) Do not worship false Gods or idols. Incest).

4) Avoid all forms of sexual immorality or impurity (particularly).

5) Do not eat a limb removed from a live animal.

6) Do not curse or blaspheme GOD.

7) Set up courts of law to promote justice and social harmony among humans.

The great Maimonides explains that any human being who faithfully observes these laws will be deemed fit to enter Heaven after the death of the physical body. This is reflected by the Rabbinic saying, "That the righteous of all nations inherit a place in Heaven."

Creation continued to grow after the flood of Noah, and the world became flawed once again. Because of the development of pagan cultures, people soon forgot about GOD and how He created the world. Instead, they prayed and relied on idols, animals, trees, and even stars. Amidst this pagan society, another hero arose: Abraham (the father of our nation), the first Patriarch. He cried out and asked GOD to save and help the world. He was blessed with a covenant that a chosen nation would come from him and help the other seventy world nations learn and remember that they were created to serve the true and living GOD.

He continued only with his son, Yitzhak (Isaac). From Yitzhak came the great sacrifice, a trait that the chosen nation earned and set them apart. They were willing to sacrifice their lives for GOD, a trait that very few can emulate.

Abraham gave many gifts to humankind. However, some of them were misused by his children. These gifts were originally wholesome wisdom but were later twisted and channeled for negative and impure uses. Below is a brief story from the Zohar (Ha Kadosh) to illustrate an example.

Rabbi Abba says, "One day, as I was traveling, I was in a particular city and met some people from India. They told me some of the ancient knowledge that is found in their books of wisdom (based on the names of the unholy side that were sent to them by Abraham to help them overcome their tendencies toward idol worship).

"I was shown one book, wherein it was written that depending on the way a person directs his will in this World, this draws down to him a special spiritual force from above. This spirit is like his desire to reach a goal he has connected himself to in this World. So, the essence of this teaching is to cleave with words, actions, and heartfelt meditation to the desired object. "If his will is directed toward something lofty and holy, he draws that thing from the spiritual realms down to himself. But, on the other hand, if he desires to cleave to the forces of impurity (i.e., ego-driven desires) and he makes this his focus of meditation, then he draws down that thing to himself from on high."

"They told me that the essence of this teaching is to cleave with words and actions and heartfelt meditation to the desired object, and by doing so, one draws down power from that side he leaves too. In this same book, I found rites and ceremonies relating to worshipping the stars and constellations, and the mantras that needed to be chanted in their worship.

"There were also instructions on how a person can concentrate his will on them to draw these forces down onto himself. "I said to them, 'My sons, these are words similar to those of the Torah. Nevertheless, you should stay well away from these books so that you are not led astray by those forms of worship and all of those negative forces mentioned there, and stray away from worshipping the Holy One, Blessed be He. All these books mislead a person."

"The ancient children of the East were wise; they inherited the wisdom that Abraham sent with the sons of his concubines, as is written, 'Abraham gave gifts to the sons of his concubines and sent them eastward [to India], away from his son Isaac, while he was still alive.' But, over time, they were drawn down many wrong paths by that wisdom."

We can now learn from the above and internalize the importance of sticking to the chain of truth (in Hebrew, Emet). Traditions and teachings were passed from Abraham to Isaac, and then to Isaac's son, Jacob. Jacob eventually had twelve sons of his own, who would later become the heads of the twelve tribes of the nation of Israel. One of them was a special boy by the name of Joseph. Yosef is also known as Yosef Hatzadek (Josef the righteous), as he was able, at 17, not to sin, along with much more. He was the next leader of Israel, and his brother, Judah (Yehuda in Hebrew). This Sageor Episode can take up an entire book itself. (More on this can be read in Genesis.) We encourage you to read independently or with a friend, family, or study partner (perhaps your local Orthodox Rabbi).

Many generations after Jacob and his family went down to Egypt, a new Pharaoh who ruled Egypt enslaved the Jews. Of course, no action that any king takes can happen contrary to the will of GOD. Not all Pharaohs were evil, but this Egyptian king made the nation of Israel his slave. His sorcerers knew and had foretold that a nation of prophets would emerge from these people, and this Pharaoh wanted control over them. One sorcerer told him that a baby boy would soon be born to liberate the Jewish people from slavery. This prompted him to issue a decree requiring the killing of all Jewish males

Newborns.

You may ask, where was GOD in all this? Well, since He had not yet revealed Himself fully, he intervened quietly and secretly with the birth of the greatest prophet ever, Moses. GOD laughed at Pharaoh's plan to murder the prophet and put the perfect plan in place so that Moses was sent right into the palace to eventually become a prince.

Moses, the greatest prophet of all, a prince of Egypt, and the humblest man of all time, needs no introduction. The entire world has heard of him and his greatness. He was soon chosen to lead the nation as he led his flock of sheep. His life is detailed in Genesis as well. We will move forward to the Giving of the Torah itself, perhaps one of the greatest moments in history.

First, it is important to note that before giving it to the Jews, GOD first offered His instructions (the Torah) to the other seventy nations of the world. They all declined for different reasons. For instance, when one nation saw the Torah forbid killing, they said, "No, we do not want that." When another saw that the Torah prohibited stealing, they replied, "No, we do not want that." They all declined the Torah to protect their own lustful and immoral addictions.

All nations had a chance to be the ones to represent the Torah (GOD's instructions) and be a "light to the nations," but they declined in a historic event filled with witnesses. So, GOD's spirit returned to this earth to teach Moses, on Mount Sinai, the secrets of creation, the aleph bet (Hebrew letters), the esoteric teachings, and the oral and written Torah. All with a purpose, a mission, perhaps the most challenging task of all time to learn, live, and teach these rules to the world.

1. Three million witnesses heard the voice of God speaking to Moses while presenting the Ten Commandments on Mount Sinai.
2. We see that many of our patriarchs and prophets have made human errors and are not perfect.
3. There is a chain of traditions passed on from Moses to this day; physical proof exists from clothing, songs, prayers, Tefillin, and more.

Our sages taught (Gemara Shabbat 146a) that when the nation of Yisroel received the Torah, their souls were cleansed of the stain caused by the sin of Adam. Thus, the people of Israel were raised to a spiritual stature equal to that of Adam before his sin. However, after signing with the Golden Calf, they sank back to the level they stood on before coming onto Mount Sinai. Moses, our great teacher, pleaded on the Jews' behalf to be forgiven; this event is filled with excellent commentaries and lessons.

We do not have enough time or space in the book to get into all those details, but we conclude that the Jews were given another chance to receive the tablets, and we will attempt to share them as well as a modern-day lesson.

4) Aseret Hadibrot

How Many Mitzvahs Are Really in the "Ten Commandments?"

By Yehuda Shurpin

The English term "Ten Commandments" is not an exact translation of the Hebrew phrase Aseret Hadibrot ("Ten Statements"). Moreover, this terminology isn't even accurate since the Aseret Hadibrot actually contains 11-15 commandments, depending on how you count.

Statements vs. Commandments

Scripture tells us that G-d communicated ten statements when He gave the Torah at Mount Sinai. G-d then engraved these statements onto two tablets and gave them to Moses to give to the people. Later, Scripture refers to them as Aseret Hadevarim, "the Ten Statements," which is more accurately rendered as the Decalogue.1 Other sources refer to them as Aseret Hadibrot, which is essentially the same thing. Nowhere in Jewish literature, from Scripture to Talmud to Kabbalah, are they ever referred to as the Ten Commandments.

A mitzvah, or commandment, is a Divine directive to perform or abstain from specific acts. An individual action item involved in an obligation or prohibition constitutes an independent mitzvah. Thus, more than one mitzvah may be included in a single paragraph or phrase of the Torah.

List of Commandments in the Decalogue

The classic 13th-century work Sefer HaChinuch, an anonymous composition, meticulously details and explains the 613 commandments according to their appearance in the Torah (based on Maimonides' enumeration of the mitzvahs). Notably, in Exodus, Sefer HaChinuch identifies a total of 14 commandments within the Decalogue:

1. To know there is a G-d

2. Not to entertain thoughts of other gods besides Him

3. Not to make an idol for yourself

4. Not to worship idols in the manner they are worshiped

5. Not to worship idols in the four ways G-d is worshiped

6. Not to take G-d's Name in vain

7. To sanctify the day of Shabbat

8. Not to do prohibited labor on the seventh day

9. To honor one's father and mother

10. Not to murder

11. Not to commit adultery

12. Not to kidnap

13. Not to testify falsely

14. Not to covet and scheme to acquire another's possession

Is the First "Commandment" a Commandment?

Some opine that the first commandment ("I am the L-rd your G-d") cannot be counted as a commandment. To quote Rabbi Chesdai Cerescas (14th century Spain):

Those who count belief in G-d as a commandment are making an error because a mitzvah, by definition, is something additional. A mitzvah cannot exist without a G-d issuing the command. Therefore, if belief in G-d is counted as a command, the person has already accepted that there is a G-d who is commanding them to believe in G-d . . . Indeed, for this reason, the Baal Halachot Gedolot (c.760 CE– c.920 CE), who was the first to formally compile a list of all the commandments in the Torah, omits belief in G-d from his list. However, the majority of those who enumerate the mitzvahs do count belief in G-d as a mitzvah. They explain that the mitzvah isn't simply the belief that G-d exists (in which case Rabbi Crescas would be correct); rather, one is commanded to believe that G-d is the most perfect and eternal Being, and He transcends all of creation.

See Is It a Mitzvah to Believe in

G-d? Other Ways of Counting

Others, notably Nachmanides, condense the clauses "Not to worship idols in the manner they are worshiped" and "Not to worship idols in the four ways we worship G-d" into a general prohibition against having other gods.

Nachmanides also opines that the prohibition against making idols is not included in the Aseret Hadibrot; rather, its primary source is in Leviticus: "You shall not turn to the worthless idols, nor shall you make molten deities for yourselves. I am the L-rd, your G-d."

Not to Covet: One or Two?

The Aseret Hadibrot appears twice in the Torah, once in Exodus and once in Deuteronomy, albeit with slight differences (see Why Two Versions of the Ten Commandments?).

In Exodus, the final instruction is not to covet (Lo tachmod). However, in Deuteronomy, the Torah adds another phrase, Lo titaveh, "You shall not desire your neighbor's house, field, etc."

While many perceive these two expressions as different aspects of the same mitzvah, Maimonides counts them as separate commandments. "Lo titaveh" refers to the prohibition of the desire, while "Lo tachmod" refers to coveting an object to the point of obtaining it. (For more on this, see "Do Not Covet"— The Prohibition against coveting another's Possessions.)

Thus, if you include Maimonides' opinion on the version of the Aseret Hadibrot in Deuteronomy, there are actually 15 mitzvahs in the Aseret Hadibrot.

What's so special about them?

Although, for the sake of clarity, we often refer to the Aseret Hadibrot as the Ten Commandments, the fact that the Torah calls them "Ten Statements" and never refers to them by the number of mitzvahs they contain underscores an essential truth. The Aseret Hadibrot aren't significant due to the specific mitzvahs within them, but rather what they represent: the giving of the entire Torah to the Jewish people.

We must know that there are 4 parts of Torah that Moshe Rabbeni gave us;

1) Written Torah, Oral Torah, Mitzvot Moshe Meh Sinai, and Esoteric secrets of Torah (known as Kabbalah). To read more about this and a great intro to kabbalah and a great translation of sefer Shomer Emunim by Rabbi Yosef Igras (alav hashalom), go to https://avinoamfraenkel.com/

5) Discipline

Discipline is the path leading one to proper, acceptable behavior. It is the discipline that enables man to control his body's physical and materialistic drives. Following the path dictated by physicality, which leads only to death, is a crooked path compared to a disciplined path, enabling man to transcend his physical dimension's control. A disciplined way of behavior, Derech Eretz is the path leading to life and eternity, a true Derech Chaim. In Brachot 5a, Rabbi Shimon Bar Yochai teaches, "GOD gave the Jewish people three presents, and each of them was only given accompanied by 'Yisurim' (difficulty). The three gifts are the Torah, the land of Israel, and the world to come."

1) As it is written (Psalms 94:12), with forward strides, Torah goes to the man disciplined by GOD (and taught His Torah).

2) As it is written (Deut. 8:5, 7), "You should know with your heart that as a man disciplines his son, GOD disciplines you." This is followed by, "For GOD brings you into a good land (Eretz Yisrael)."

3) The World to come, as it is written (Prov. 6:23), "For a mitzvah is a lamp, and Torah is light, and reproofs of discipline are the way of life."

These things were explicitly given and accompanied by discipline because each is sanctified and elevated. The land of Israel is holy and special, having in it more wisdom and spirituality than any other land, as evidenced by "the air in Israel makes one wise" (Baba Batra 158b) and the occurrence of prophecy taking place only in Eretz Israel. The Torah is not rooted in the physical (while human intellectual disciplines are) as purely divine wisdom. Therefore, the world to come is particularly sanctified and elevated, having no eating, drinking, or any physical activity.

There is a progression from something essentially a material thing, the land of Israel, which has a spiritual dimension, to the Torah, which requires a material world for its performance and is studied by human beings. Yet, it is a spiritual reality, through Olam Habah, which has no material dimension, being purely transcendent and spiritual. It is for this reason that these three are all called (matanot) gifts. A gift is given to a person who does not have access to it on his own and who does not emanate from within him. Instead, it is given to him by a completely independent source. Since man exists in a physical body, and these three things are divine and holy, transcending the physical, there is no way they can develop from within man.

They must be GIVEN to man from an outside source, by GOD. It requires discipline and limits to the physical dimension of man to enable man to assimilate the holy and divine presence. The Maharal elaborates on this point in chapter two of Netivot Ha Yeshorim.

This gives us an insight into the difficulties encountered continuously by people trying to make Aliya. Rabbi Shaya Karlinsky, Dean of Darche Noam Institutions, taught, "For Eretz Yisrael to properly absorb a Jew, and for a Jew to properly absorb the special nature of Eretz Yisrael, the person's relationship to Israel cannot be built on a purely materialistic pursuit. People coming to Israel to raise their standard of living usually do not make it. This, because Jews were always at the forefront of building healthy and strong economies in nearly every society in which they found themselves.

It appears that the Jewish relationship with Israel is not purely an economic and physical one. Even the early settlers who drained swamps, fought malaria, and built the land upon a physical and agricultural level did so with tremendous 'YISURIM,' discipline, and physical suffering." It can indeed be said that they transcended their physical natures in their quest to gain a portion of the land of Israel.

As noted above, a great sacrifice is essential for growth; therefore, you must take hits in life. There will be ups and downs along your beautiful journey, so to maximize your learning, we recommend that you now search for a teacher or master to guide you. There is only so much this book can do to help you, and at some point, you will need face-to-face interaction with a master. If you are wondering where in the world you can find one, Below are some pointers. Do not forget:

In the path that man wishes to go, GOD will guide him, and along with your prayers, the path will be more visible. Pray for a good teacher, and with divine help, you will find one. There is a wealth of information that depends on the person, which can take months or years to grasp. Therefore, we suggest you take a break or, for some of you, take a vacation before you decide to move forward.

6) Choosing a Teacher or Master

As the Mishnah/Gemara suggests (in Taanit), we must choose a teacher who has Derech Eretz, i.e., character traits that are kind and refined.

Therefore, learn only from those scholars that are kind and caring, with a solid character, or as the great sage, Avtalyon, would say: "Sages, be careful with your words, lest you be punished with exile, and you will be exiled to the place of the bad waters, and your students who come after you will drink, and the name of heaven will be profaned." (Avot, 1:11)

Rambam explains that Avtalyon cautions teachers not to teach ambiguously, enabling students to understand heretical interpretations of their master's lectures. For example, he cites the well-known story in which a misinterpretation of Antigonos Sochos' teachings helped launch the Sadducee movement. Antignos taught (Avot 1:3) that religious people should not serve GOD as does a servant looking for a reward. Tzadok and Baitus heard this and reasoned that only someone who does not believe in the existence of a future reward would teach such a doctrine.

Thus, they initiated movements denying life after death and future compensation for our actions here on earth. Josephus confirms this account of the Sadducees' denial of a world to come (Antiquities of the Jews, 18:1:4), proving their rejection of the rabbinic tradition. Since biblical accounts of reward and punishment focus on a material desert rather than on the next world (see Abrabanel's commentary at the beginning of Bechukotai for a survey of explanations for this phenomenon), the Sadducees rejected the oral tradition of a world to come.

Rabbi Avi Weinstein explains that this teaches us something quite important: even correct messages require scrutiny for potential damage. Antigonus taught a basic idea, calling for idealistic motivation instead of reducing religious life to a practical and pragmatic affair. However, he did not fully appreciate how students might hear his words. Instead, they speculated that he shifted attention away from reward because no such reward exists. Had Antigonus expected this negative fallout, he might have emphasized the idealistic motivation while simultaneously affirming his belief in the afterlife and divine justice: "Sages, be careful with your words."

The Abarbanel suggests that the imagery of exile refers to national exile and the resulting intermingling with other peoples and cultures. Such intermingling has enabled Jews to learn great things from other people. However, it also opens up the danger of students looking to restructure Judaism to fit in with or be compatible with the latest fads in broader society. Such students may search for any statement of their teachers that will enable the grafting of currently popular but incompatible elements into the Jewish religion. Therefore, teachers need to clearly state which outside cultural areas deserve respect and which require forceful rejection. The culture clash demands even greater care for language on behalf of our instructors.

If you want to learn more about the chain of events, time, space, and more, we encourage you to keep reading, learning, and growing! Many people have asked the question: What happens after the body dies? Is there more? What is next after our physical body leaves this earth?

7) Life after life?

I will not get into this too much because this is not the point of this book. Still, it is essential to touch on it briefly to realize that our time on this earth is very precious, every moment of every hour. It is an opportunity to do well and serve as a light to others. Once our time passes on this earth, we no longer have a chance to do righteous acts and accrue merit for ourselves any longer; we lose our free choice and ability to earn merits.

We move on to be judged according to our past actions and our work in this world. If our actions on Earth were good, then many sages have taught of seven levels of heaven in which we ascend according to our merits. The seven levels of Heaven are what we may call the "holding stage" of paradise, where we can learn more Torah and get prepared for the final return to the Messianic area. If we do not do our job, then, unfortunately, there is a return to Earth (reincarnation) to take another shot at life.

The final return will be the long-awaited Messianic era, where the world is filled with a complete understanding of GOD's perfect teaching and complete and total knowledge of His ways as they relate to humanity. It will be a balanced and ideal rule under the one true GOD. It will be His rules "set into play."

In the world of Judaism, as mentioned in particular by the Kabbalah, when a person goes on to the next world (passes away), his soul can come back in another body or form to fix the things he messed up in his previous life.

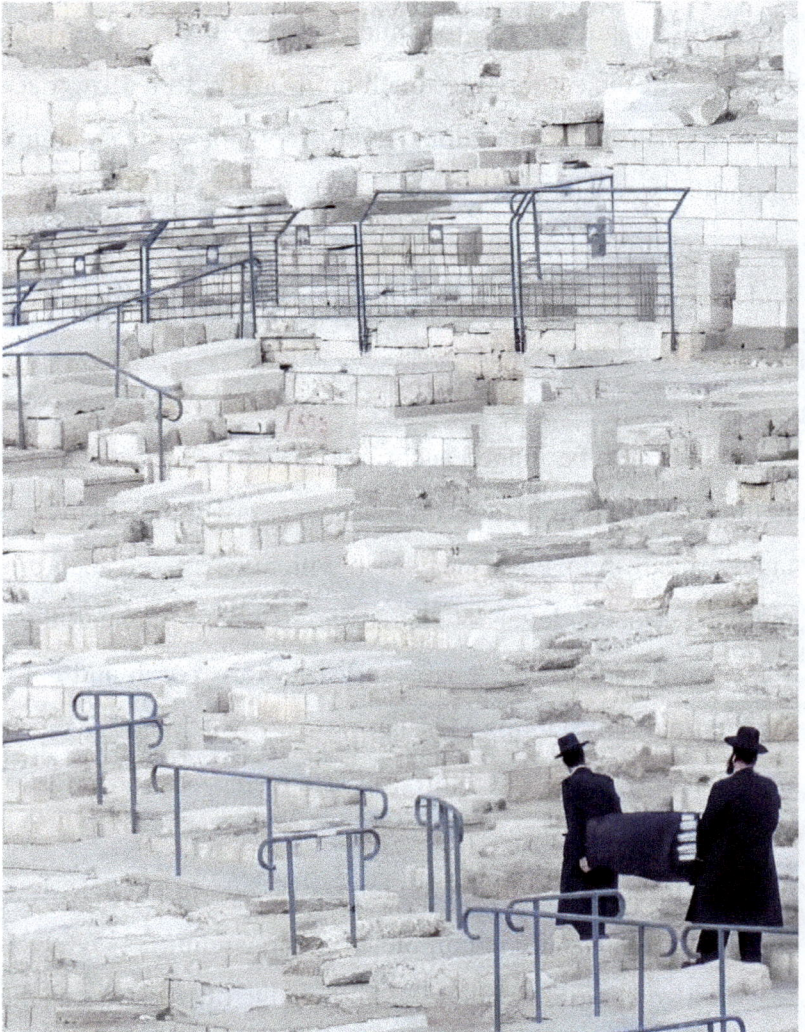

Such a returning soul is engaged in a process called gilgul neshamot. According to the Jewish sages, the purpose of such a return is to aid in Tikkun, or "repairing/healing of the world." Hence, the individual's "purpose-driven" return to earth is part of a greater cosmic hope for the eventual revitalization and restoration of the universe.

What Is the Point of All This?

The objective is to fix humankind's evil choices and bring perfection back to the world. Until that happens, people leave and enter this world. Many enter a different level of heaven (7 levels), some Gan Eden, and some Gehinnom (for a spiritual cleansing). More about this can be read in various books, such as The Afterlife (the Jewish View), Where Are We Headed? by Jonathan Morgenstern, and Rabbi Sholom Kamenetsky.

To sum up, you want to learn and practice Emunah (faith) or gratitude through faith and hope. This can take years to practice, but when we can see that every little detail that happens to us is not only from GOD but is for our very good, we can get closer to the life of Emunah. This can be difficult; for instance, a minor scratch on your car, a bruise on your body, traffic, a delay in the airport, your friend or wife taking longer than expected to get ready, etc.

If we can make each event in our lives for the best, we can live happier. I am not saying to be negligent or to be late to places. I am saying to do your best. Once you have done your best and things are not in your control (you can hand it over to GOD), all the outcomes are for your very best to learn and grow from.

Many take losses and difficulties in life way too hard or negatively, but if we can see these moments as a chance for learning and growth or accept them at face value, it can be the best attitude. You might wonder why so many Chassidim (perhaps the famous Chabad or Breslov Jews) dance and sing so often. Because they have practiced these concepts of faith for so long and engraved them into their inner beings.

Once you realize that all that happens outside your will is not only not in your hands but also the best thing for you, you will sing and dance as well. You know you have a loving father who loves you and rotates the world all for you! You would dance and sing and be thankful as well! It is a state of mind that takes practice. Sometimes, the clapping of the hands or singing a little melody can help remind you of this.

While we are still on this Earth, gratitude to our Creator has powerful possibilities. Anyone can become greater than what they currently are. You can be a hero, but are you willing to take the hits to get there and keep learning and advancing? The choice is yours. We understand how pursuing such vices as lust, honor, jealousy, and hatred can easily take a person out of this world, out of the "Garden State of mind." So, take care of your soul by practicing compassion, love, and respect for one another and having a fear of GOD.

8) The Kabbalah

Kabbalah is our ancient Jewish mystical teachings that teach the most profound insights into the essence of GOD, His interaction with the world, and the purpose of creation.

The Kabbalah and its teachings are no less than the Law and are an integral part of the Torah. They are traced back to Avraham Avinu, our patriarch, who wrote the Sefer Ha Yetzirah book for formation. It is the first book that mentions a system of ten lights called Sephirot.
The Kabbalah itself teaches that its study is an essential method for helping to advance the final Messianic redemption and perfect the world.

Maimonides gives an example of this: He asks us to imagine a line of a thousand blind people going on a journey led at the head of the line by at least one person who can see. They can still be sure that they are going in the right direction. They will not fall into any snares or traps in their path since they follow someone who can see. But if the one person who can see is absent, they will undoubtedly stumble over every obstacle laid in their path, and they will all fall into a dark pit.

A brief History of Kabbalah (from the book Arizal, Prince of Kabbalist by Rabbi Raphael Afilalo) Approximately 1750 BCE, Avraham Avinu Approximately 240 CE, Israel, with Rabbi Shimon Bar Yochai: 1200-1300, with the new era of printing, a book of Zohar is found by Rabbi Moshe De Leon in Spain. Provence in France, Gerona in Spain, and Worms in Germany formed three of the main centers of Kabbalah during that period.

Prominent Kabbalists include Rabbi Itzhak the Blind, Rabbi Ezra of Gerona, and Rabbi El'azar of Worms. 1500, Tsfat Kabbalist. After the expulsion of Spain in 1492, some important Spanish Kabbalists came to Tzfat, Israel. Rabbi Moshe Cordovero (1522-1570) was the founder of the Kabbalah Academy of Tzfat. His great works are Tomer Deborah, Pardes Rimonim, and Or Yakar. Soon to be the Golden Era of Kabbalah.

Rabbi Yosef Karo also had a revelation of a Maggid (celestial mentor) who disclosed to him deep Kabbalah secrets. During this generation, Rabbi Yitzchak Luria Ashkenazi, the Arizal (1534–1574), was born in Jerusalem and soon became the "Prince of the Kabbalah." He explained the main concepts of Kabbalah. He is the author of the corpus Ets Haim, Kitve HaAri, which contains all his works in the style of Sha'are (entrances) and is today the major reference in Kabbalah.
Rabbi Haim Vital (1542-1620) is primarily known as the leading student and writer of the teachings of the Arizal. 1700, Hasidic Movement The Hasidic period began with the Baal Shem Tov (1698-1760), who founded the Hasidic movement. He declared the whole universe, mind, and matter to be a manifestation of GOD and that

whoever maintains that his life is worthless is in error. Rabbi Nachman of Breslov (1772-1811), great-grandson of the Baal Shem Tov, gave great importance to Devekut (attachment to GOD) and our joy! Some of his main works are Likutei Moharan, Tikkun Haklali, and his well-known stories and fables.

Rabbi Shnuer Zalman of Liadi (1745-1813), the Baal Ha Tanya, founder of the Chabad Lubavitch movement. He studied under the Maggid of Mezrich and the writings of Ari and composed the Tanya. European Masters 1700, Europe

Rabbi Moshe Luzzato (Ramchal, 1707-1746) lived in Italy and Amsterdam. It is said that when he was only fourteen, he already knew all the Kabbalah of the Arizal by heart, and nobody even knew about it.

Rabbi Elyahu of Vilna, the Gaon of Vilna (1720-1797), born in Lithuania, is considered one of the greatest Torah scholars and Kabbalists.

Sephardic Masters

Rabbi Shalom Sharabi, the Rashash (1720-1777).

After leaving Yemen, although he was already known in his country as a Kabbalist, he kept his abilities hidden in the Land of Yisrael. He was hired as a Shamash in Beit El Yeshiva, the main center of Kabbalah study in Israel.

In this role, he stayed as anonymous as he could. He took a job (Shamash) to keep the books in order and serve drinks and hot tea! In addition, he would leave notes of unanswered questions in books to help students. His prominent publications are Siddur HaRashash, the main prayer book used today by Kabbalists, and Rehovot HaNahar.

Rabbi Yaacov Abehsera (1808-1880), born in Morocco, was a kabbalist renowned for his piety and performing miracles. Some of his main works are Makhsof HaLavan and Pithe 'Hotmail. Also from Morocco was Rabbi Haim Ben 'Atar Or Hachaim (1696-1743). The Bal Shem Tov was convinced that the Or Hachaim was the Mashiah of that generation. His main work is the commentary on the Torah, Or Hahaim, by Rabbi Yosef Haim Ben Ish 'Hai (1834-1909). Born in Iraq, he was a prolific author who explained the Halakot (laws) on the Kabbalistic level in an accessible language.

The Last Kabbalist, 1900, Israel One of the most important Kabbalists was Rabbi Yehudah Ashlag (1886-1955). His main work is the translation of the Zohar from Aramaic to Hebrew, called Hasulam (The Ladder). Other important Kabbalists are Rabbi Israel Abe'hetsera Baba Sali (1890-1984), Rabbi Yehudah Tzvi Brandwein (1904-1969), Rabbi Avraham Yitzhak Ha Cohen Kook (1865-1935), Rabbi Yehudah Fatiyah (1859-1942), Rabbi Itshak Kaduri (1898-2006), and others.

Each of these great scholars and Kabbalists brought their explanations and innovations to this marvelous gift. To study Kabbalah without first building a strong foundation is like studying astrophysics before you know simple subtraction and multiplication. We advise first learning to work on your character (Middot), as this is a prerequisite to learning Torah. Once you are past building your character and keeping mitzvot such as kosher, Shabbat, and basic Halachot, it can be considered touching upon cleansing the soul.

A great guide to Torah study can be found in a book called Crossing the Narrow Bridge by Rabbi Chaim Kramer. See Appendix A. The seder limud should be planned with one's rabbi. The subjects that apply are the Torah with Rashi, prophets, writings, Shulchan Aruch, Mishna, Talmud, Mussar, ethics, and Chassidut.

This book is a must to build a healthy, strong foundation and plan for growth. Understand there will be ups and downs; stay positive. Hidbodedut (speaking to GOD in your own language throughout the day in nature or in a car, etc.). This is a must in today's world. Once you have advanced in learning, which can take years (depending on the time you put in), there is an excellent set of books called Hok Le Israel. Hok L'Yisrael is a compiled daily study guide on the Weekly Torah Portion, including sections of Torah, Prophets, Scriptures, Mishna, Talmud, Zohar, Jewish law, and Jewish thought. It is said that the Holy Ari of Tzfat designated most of the selections of Hok. The custom nowadays amongst many Jews is to study the Hok L'Yisrael every day after the morning prayers. It permits one to study, in a short time, all the different sections of both the written and oral Torah.

It is said that Ari used to say it while still wearing his tallit and tefillin. (Mishna Berura 155: 1, 3. Kaf Hachayim ibid., Ot 3.) There is also a tradition that the Chida (Rabbi Chaim Yosef David Azulai) helped edit the Hok to make it more user-friendly.

9) Israel and Eretz Yisrael

We are blessed and so thankful that today we have the state of Israel. There are numerous miracles taking place daily in the holiest of lands, but just like a loving father must rebuke his children out of love, we must inform you of a few historical facts. Firstly, it is important to understand that Israel is blessed and is the Jewish people's land. A place where the light will shine to the world, a place where two of the Beit Hamikdash (holy temples) once stood, and a place where the third and final temple will be built. However, to get to that goal, we must understand what has been going on in Israel. In addition, we need to solve what we can do to make it better and bring redemption closer.

The modern state of Israel has been and is currently influenced by the conservative and reform movements. These groups have poured in millions of dollars to distance Jews from Orthodox Judaism. Take it from a source I got for several middle-class Israelis who have been there through the wars; they have admitted that many politicians take money for various agendas that distance Jews from the Creator.

Conservatism and reform movements have distanced thousands of Jews from the Torah. The Zionists, although many have righteous intentions, are also uprooting Jewish children from our religion.

Below is a piece from The Midrash Says, Bamidbar; Parashat Pinchas, by Rabbi Moshe Weisman: "When religious war orphans who survived concentration camps emigrated to Eretz Yisrael, the youth leaders, upon instructions from the various agencies, gave them non-kosher foods, i.e., ham and pigs raised in the leftist kibbutzim. They slaughtered chickens in front of the children to demonstrate they were not killed according to Jewish law. Many of the liberal Zionists also did not allow the saying of kaddish for their murdered parents, whose last wish before being sent to the gas chambers was that their children should grow up to be Torah Jews.

Against their will, they placed them in irreligious schools and kibbutzim. They trained these children to despise their parents and forebears and assimilated them into life in modern Israeli society. These Zionists also forcibly prevented tens of thousands of religious immigrants from oriental countries from fulfilling the mitzvot. When the Sephardic children arrived, the Youth Aliyah leaders snipped off their payot (side locks).

They taught them that Shabbat and kashrut were antiquated relics of the "old country, no longer relevant in modern society." Many immigrant families were placed against their will in irreligious communities instead of settling in religious cities of their choice, such as Bnei Brak in Jerusalem.

Their children were forced to attend the local irreligious schools, and any attempt to give the children a Torah education was swiftly opposed and thwarted. All statements made above are amply supported by documentation.

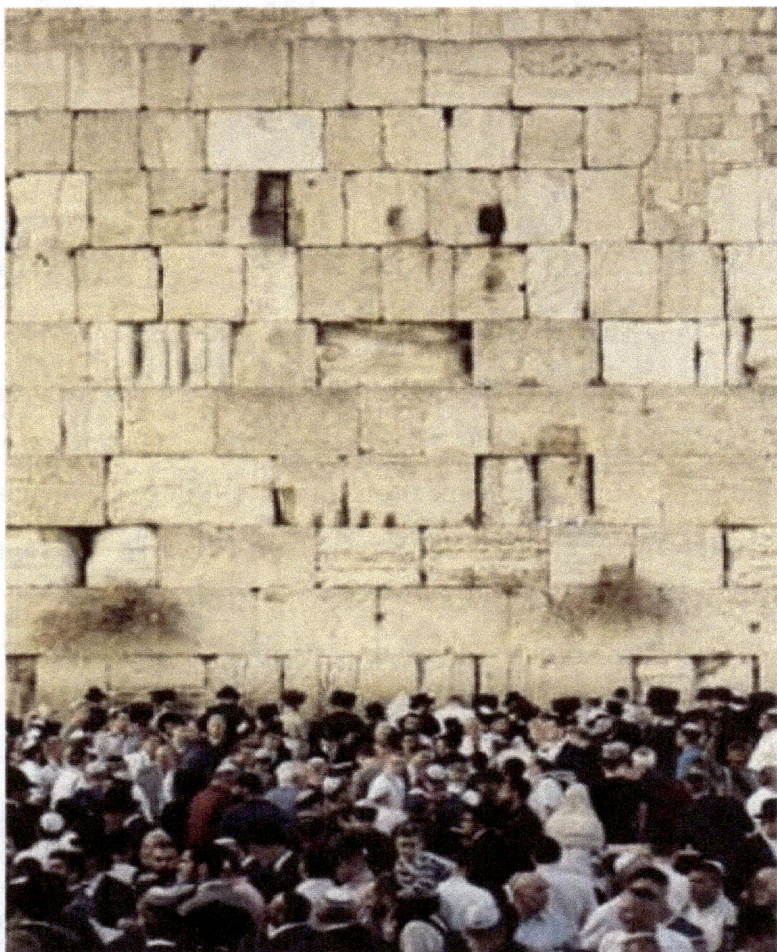

114.

The process of weaning Jewish youth from their rightful spiritual heritage continues today in the majority of schools and educational institutions of modern-day Israel.

Simultaneously, rabbis and spiritual leaders worldwide ironically rally their congregants to aid organizations like those described above. The rupture over the greatness of the mitzvah comes in lending moral and financial support to those who mislead Jews. Rather, they ought to be appealing for fundraising to establish and maintain the yeshivot in every town of Eretz Yisrael and wherever Jews live.

Suppose we fail to contemplate that a fate far more tragic than physical death has befallen and continues to threaten thousands of unfortunate Jewish souls. In that case, we demonstrate that we are insensitive to genuine Torah values. This would teach that spiritual death is equivalent to but is more tragic than physical death. If we support those organizations that tear away Jews from Torah, we too are guilty," Rabbi Moshe Weisman.

Well, it is not so surprising that this piece came from the weekly portion of the righteous and zealous Pinchas. His soul is somehow connected to the soul of Elijah, the prophet (Elijah Hanavi); both were enthusiastic about God in keeping the Torah. Yet, in my humble opinion and also from reading the book Eliyahu Hanavi by Avraham Yom Tov Rotenberg, I have learned that it is just as important, if not more, to not only be devoted to GOD but to

Be zealous as well about his children, or our fellow Jewish brothers and sisters.

This is where we once again emphasize the importance of having a master teacher, such as a Rebbe/Rabbi/Rav. Someone who can help you make unbiased, life-changing decisions. A quick sports analogy: if you may, some call it the "calls outside the lines."

For instance, if you are in the heat of the moment or game, your passions/ emotions (anger, fury) can quickly take over your mind and influence your decision-making. It is necessary to take a timeout or have a coach run a play. This can help one get their mind back into focus and or heart where it should be. Well, in our case, break down the law (halacha). We must pray to find a spiritual leader who has learned in the great chain from our ultimate Rabbi (Moshe Rabenu).

Before we begin to judge other Jews, we must first learn what is allowed and not allowed. In addition, it is crucial to start to understand that many Jews have never received a chance to learn the Torah properly and do not know any better. Therefore, it is necessary to be zealous for the right reasons and be patient with many of our brothers and sisters, as we do not know what they have gone through or are currently going through. God loves all his children, and he knows our shortcomings. We do not need to remind Him of them.

The famous Chair of Elyahu Hanavi is present in every Brit Millah. Well, if we can connect the zealousness of Pinchas/Eliyahu Hanavi, we can see why he comes to witness every single Brit Millah; to remind us all how amazing the Jewish people are! We must

Remind ourselves how incredible the Jewish people are and educate them in a kind and loving manner.

Begin to educate other Jews to return to the path of the Torah and steer them away from reform and conservative (or watered-down Torah) and show them the absolute truth in a loving way. With love, patience, and education, the modern-day state of Israel will transform to become Eretz Yisrael, and the greatest kingdom ever will reign there for eternity. You're Doing Great!

Now that you have come this far, learning the history of creation and our purpose on Earth. We encourage you to live the life of a winner, one who never gives up or takes their eyes off the prize in the race of life. This next section was added as the last part of the book during the Virus of 2020; with many people in sorrow and a loss of faith, we decided to share some wisdom and strengthen ourselves during these very challenging times. So, before we begin the section, I want to introduce two crucial concepts that I believe will help give you confidence, clarity, and faith during these very challenging times. First are the 13 principles of our faith, and second are the 3 cardinal sins.

To understand the 13 principles, we must first know where we came from and where we were headed. The Jewish nation has battled many evil leaders and empires, and some of our holy days reflect this: Hanukkah (Greeks), Purim (Persians), Romans (during the 2nd temple era), and so much more. Whether dealing with the virus or "pandemic," an evil scheme by a group attempting to create

Population, health, and currency control—we must stay strong in our faith and unite as we have in the past. Now even more so.

Here is a passage from the world-famous writer, publisher, and entrepreneur, Mr. Mark Twain.

On the Jews

His contributions to the world's list of great names in literature, science, art, music, finance, medicine, and abstruse learning are also very out of proportion to the weakness of his numbers. He has made a marvelous fight in this world in all ages and has done it with his hands tied behind him. He could be vain of himself and be excused for it.

The Egyptians, the Babylonians, and the Persians rose, filled the planet with sound and splendor, then faded to dream stuff and passed away; the Greeks and Romans followed and made a vast noise, and they were gone; other people have sprung up and held their torch high for a time, but it burned out, and they sit in twilight now and have vanished.

The Jew saw them all, survived them all, and is now what he always was, exhibiting no decadence, no infirmities of age, no weakening of his parts, no slowing of his energies, and no dulling of his alert but aggressive mind.

All things are mortal but the Jews; all other forces pass, but he remains. What is the secret of his immortality? September 1897

(Quoted in The National Jewish Post & Observer, June 6, 1984) I would like to reiterate to all Jews to practice and share perhaps a secret to our existence and something we must implement daily to help us win this battle to restore faith and harmony in the world.

10) Principles of Faith

Rabbi Moshe ben Maimon compiled what he refers to as the Shloshah Asar Ikkarim, the "Thirteen Fundamental Principles" of the Jewish faith, as derived from the Torah. Maimonides refers to these thirteen principles of faith as "the fundamental truths of our religion and its very foundations."

1. Belief in the existence of the Creator, who is perfect in every manner of existence and is the Primary Cause of all that exists.

2. The belief in GOD's absolute and unparalleled unity.

3. The belief in GOD's non-corporeality, nor that He will be affected by any physical occurrences, such as movement, rest, or dwelling.

4. The belief in GOD's eternity.

5. The imperative to worship GOD exclusively and no foreign false gods.

6. The belief that GOD communicates with man through prophecy.

7. The belief in the primacy of the prophecy of Moses, our teacher.

8. The belief in the divine origin of the Torah.

9. The belief in the immutability of the Torah.

10. The belief in GOD's omniscience and providence.

11. The belief in divine reward and retribution.

12. The belief in the arrival of the Messiah and the messianic era.

13. The belief in the resurrection of the dead.

We must know that if we protect these 13, they will protect us. This means living by these with our whole hearts and educating others about them. In addition to the 13 principles of faith, it is crucial to share another element of our survival: the observance and respect of the 3 cardinal sins.

Perhaps another secret to our eternal survival and why the Jews have found a life worth living is that we have three areas in which one must sacrifice his life. The three cardinal sins are best explained by an Aish rabbi. Maimonides writes that if a person were to say to a Jew, "Violate one of the commandments or I will kill you," the Jew should violate the commandment and not be killed, since the Torah says, "You shall observe My decrees and My laws so that you shall live by them." The inference from the words "live by them" is that you shall not "die by them!"

This, however, does not apply to three mitzvahs:

1) Murder

2) Forbidden sexual relations

3) Worship of other gods.

(Maimonides—Foundations of the Torah 5:2)

MURDER

Imagine the case: Mike says to Dave, "Either you kill that person, or I will kill you." The law states that Dave must allow himself to be killed rather than kill the other person. The reason is logical, in the language of the Talmud: "What makes you think your blood is redder than his? Perhaps his blood is redder!" Or, in other words, "How can you judge between your life and his? Perhaps he is worthier than you!" Since it is impossible to know who the "better Jew" is, one must let the circumstances play out without killing the other person. (Yoma 82b)

This logic applies even if Mike were to say to the inhabitants of a Jewish town, "Give me one Jew to kill, or if you do not, I will kill all of you." Since it is impossible to decide whose blood is the "least red," the town must not butcher anyone to be killed. (Maimonides, Yesodei HaTorah 5:5).

FORBIDDEN SEXUAL RELATIONS

Someone must allow himself to be killed rather than be involved in forbidden sexual relations because the Torah compares rape to murder.

(Deuteronomy 22:26, Talmud Yoma 82a)

IDOL WORSHIP: The gods come from a verse in the Shema: "You shall love your GOD with all your heart, WITH ALL YOUR SOUL, and with all your possessions" (Deuteronomy 6:5). In other words, you should love GOD so much that you are willing to give up your life to serve him (Talmud Yoma 82a).

The reason why loving GOD with all your soul applies explicitly to the worship of other Gods is that the belief that "GOD is one," the Creator and Controller of everything, is the basis for all of Judaism. We can see from above the incredible greatness of the mitzvah of sanctifying GOD's name and the traits that exist deep down in the soul of every Jew.

Living by the above principles and rules, we can see that Jews have a life worth living with real meaning. No matter what may happen to our loved ones or to us, if we live according to the will of God, He will bring us back stronger and happier, with all our loved ones, in a better world at the right time.

11) Pandemic or Pandemic of 2020

GOD and the Virus/Plague: Rabbi Benjamin Blech The virus of 2020 is now officially a "global pandemic." Suddenly, we find ourselves smitten by a plague of biblical severity. Passover asks us to remember the ten plagues that GOD sent to the Egyptians. With the help of the Bible, we know the purpose behind these afflictions. GOD had a plan. Egyptian suffering had meaning. What makes our contemporary anguish so particularly unbearable is its seeming incomprehensibility. In the age of prophets, there would have been an effort to discern some divine message in this global tragedy.

Today, we somehow assume that scientific knowledge precludes the possibility of including GOD as part of the management of the universe. After all, who can argue with Louis Pasteur and Robert Koch, who, in the latter half of the 19th century, proved the germ theory of disease—that "pathogens too small to see without magnification are the true cause of illness"? Thus, germs are the villains, and viruses are the sole reasons for the presence of diseases that determine whether we live or die.

I dare to ask: Does not believing in GOD demand that we merge the germ theory of disease with the conviction of faith in a supreme being who actually decides where, when, and how far a virus can spread?

When we are directed by doctors to wash our hands, we must do so according to Torah law. Please understand exactly what I am saying. Maimonides, long ago, made clear that we must ensure our good health. We cannot simply rely on GOD; GOD has made us his partners in our quest for longevity.

Hygiene is a mitzvah; it is an obligation. Taking care of our bodies is a spiritual requirement akin to protecting our souls. As we make clear every year on Rosh Hashanah and Yom Kippur, when our fate is sealed, the ultimate decision of life or death remains with the Almighty. That is why I am amazed by the countless suggestions for how to counter and cope with the virus. We hear so little of the word God and the possibility that this global pandemic brings a profound divine message. I am no prophet, but here is a thought that I think is worth considering and taking to heart.

Every parent knows that one of the most obvious responses to a child's misbehavior is what is commonly known as a "timeout." The child is temporarily restricted from enjoying pleasurable activities. The child has their everyday life disrupted. The child is encouraged to reflect upon their disobedience. Is it too much to consider that our world continues to sink ever lower in our commitment to virtue and that GOD responded with a virus that has forced millions into a "timeout" of quarantine and seclusion?

The Ten Commandments are the biblical source of the most basic system of ethical and moral behavior. They represent the primary justification for our continued existence on earth, and the commentators took note of a remarkable number. In the original Hebrew language, where the commandments were inscribed by GOD, there are precisely 620 letters on the two tablets. 620 would seem to be a number with no particular theological significance. However, it would have been perfect and readily comprehensible if there were precisely 613 letters in the 10 Commandments. Those are the number of mitzvot given to the Jewish people in the Torah.

Moreover, the 10 Commandments are the principles inherent in all Jewish law. So, what is the meaning of the 620 letters? The rabbis explained. While the number of mitzvot for Jews is 613, the number seven represents universal law—what is commonly referred to as the seven laws of the descendants of Noah, required as a minimum for all of mankind. 620 is the sum of 613 and 7, the totality of divine guidance for the Jews and the rest of the world. The word "plague" comes from the Latin word "plaga." The commentary does not end there.

620 is the gematria, the numerical value, of an important Hebrew word, Keter, which means crown. A Keter crown is placed on top of every Torah scroll. The symbolism is obvious. The crown above the Torah demonstrates the relationship of the 10 Commandments to the rest of the Torah. From the 10 in number of letters numbered 620, we have the principles that subsequently found expression in the entirety of the

Torah. The Keter crown is the most powerful symbol of our connection with GOD. The word they gave to the plague comes from the Latin word for crown.

Nonetheless, we must listen to the good doctors and rabbis to take care of our health. When we speak and think well, the world will be good. We must take upon ourselves more sanctity, or, in Hebrew, the Kedusha. When we think and speak with Kedusha, so shall the upper worlds return the Kedusha down to us. Finally, we hope that while you are reading this, the "plague" will be over, and you will have taken it upon yourselves to be closer to GOD and in a state of mind of Torah, chessed, and mitzvot.

As my friend Rabbi Vosoghi put it, "King Hizkiyau once had a book that had all the remedies to all the sicknesses in the world. One of the best things he did was hide that book. Why, you may ask? Well, because every time there was a sickness or a plague, people went straight to the book.

They worshiped the book instead of digging down deep and praying to GOD. They wanted a quick fix, a segulah." Therefore, we must use this time to increase our prayers, work on all the areas we need to (each to his own), and focus on our relationship with GOD, along with our fellow man (wife, kids, friend, etc.). Lastly, we will end this with a response from the Gaon Rebbe Shlomo Yehudah Beeri Shalita, or his nickname, the "Yanuka":

"People think they know who HaKadosh Baruch Hu is and what Torah is, and then, Hashem suddenly does something that no one can process, shaking up the order of Creation," Rav Shlomo Yehudah explains. "Once we understand that we have no grasp of the Creator and begin to serve Him with terminus and with awe, no longer being so sure we have all the answers and instead looking with respect for everyone simply because they have a Tzelem Elokim, then perhaps this pandemic will be annulled, b'ezras Hashem."

He believes that the violation of the Tzelem Elokim through lashon hara and sinas chinam is even hinted at in the lockdown rules. "The isolation period for those who have come in contact with coronavirus is 14 days, like the isolation for the metzora who speaks lashon hara," the Yanuka clarifies. "The metzora had to sit alone outside the camp, the quintessential social distancing. So, our work now is to draw closer to the soul of the other, to feel with the other, and to be aware of his needs.

And that," says Rav Shlomo Yehudah, "is the way forward, as it appears to me." He has many lectures about finding the good in others, respecting your Rabbanim, and more on his online channel. He is a true gem, and we recommend listening to his classes, which now have English subtitles. For those music fans, he plays miraculous melodies that allow you to cling to the creator, which are on the channel as well.

12) Final Battle vs. Amalek

The world seems to be in a battle of "control." But, of course, it is Hashem's world, and only the arrogance, ego, and greed of some men think they can take control of the world (from financial to population control; see more here (https://www.rodefshalom613.org/)). What initially seemed like a conspiracy theory to many appears to be more evident with the rise and fear of people pushing for a virus.

How can a house of prayer get fined when a stadium or movie theater is allowed to open? Of course, we must take care of our health and bodies, but the extreme measures seem unreal and manipulated. There are plenty of stories out there; we do not need to even mention them. An analogy: one of my rabbis, Harav Ha Gaon Eliyahu Netaneli Shlita, said if it were not for Haman, we would not have Purim, not for the Greeks' Hanukkah, and of course, without Pharaoh, perhaps no Exodus.

So, we see how many mitzvot and good things come from what seems "evil" in the world, so fear not. We should fear Hashem and serve him as best we can. He is playing with the puppets of the world and pulling all the strings. It is interesting to learn and note a view from Rav Avraham Baruch, who said from a Tzadik Nistar (hidden Tzadik), we have the power to make a choice and a change. He says our last and final battle will be dependent upon 3 things:

1. Teshuva (see The Comeback/Return section)

2. Smart devices (phones and laptops), which we also explained, must have filters, and we should be ready to sacrifice smart devices if the situation demands that it get to that point.

3. Women's Modesty: Perhaps the last and maybe most important point is the modesty of women.

We all must accept that a woman must feel beautiful, and this is very important for her. According to the master kabbalist, the Arizal, the souls of the last generation before Mashiach's arrival are reincarnations of the souls of the generation of Exodus. Just as then it was in the merit of the women's faith that the Israelites were redeemed, so, too, it will be in the merit of the righteous women of our generation and their unwavering belief in the Redemption that we will be redeemed once again. This must be done correctly and with respect. A woman must be modest about her actions, speech, and clothing.

She should limit unnecessary talks with men and not wear tight clothing (but of course not baggy clothing either); she should look and feel beautiful, but in a modest fashion. She should not wear super bright and eye-catching colors, and her speech and behavior should be modest. She should not wear pants. Skirts should be above her.
Knees. There is no heater for wigs; we must follow our sages and take heed in this top and cover with a mitpachat. This is a super hard test, but worth all the sacrifice. To read more about this topic, there is a sefer called Adorned with Dignity, and there is also great material on www.malachiei26.com. She should wear shirts covering her elbows

and take the advice of a righteous Rebbetzin or a woman familiar with these laws. If you see a woman wearing a wig, pray for her and also look at your own sins and repent. Bal Shem Tov teaches that the world is a mirror; if we see sin, it's on us more than them. Pray for others and see good in them; love them, and teach them proper ways. This will help lead to Geula (Redemption) with Rachamim (with Mercy).

We must stop blaming people, including presidents, social groups, doctors, etc. We must start taking responsibility, look in the mirror, and make a change. God wants us to wake up and improve our character and start doing mitzvot.

GOD is running the show, and these "world leaders" are his puppets; we must each change ourselves. Look at the mirror, not the media, for your answers. No more excuses or blaming (that is what losers do); be a winner, take responsibility, and become better. Even a little each day will help; you will see things change for the better.

The second Beit Hamikdash was destroyed because of baseless hatred (Sinat Hinam in Hebrew). Below is a lesson we can also learn and grow with. When we get to Heaven (Shamayim) after 120, the Zohar says one of the questions we will be asked is if we crowned our friend. Basically, did we treat our friends/loved ones/all Jews like A king? Did we have their back? Did we support them when they were down? Did we hurt their feelings? Did we respect and love them for who they are? How will we respond? Our beloved Beit Hamigdash was destroyed because of Sinat Chinam! We must wake up and open our hearts and minds...

The rectification is Ahavat Chinam! It is time to wake up! Mask or no mask, let's stop judging negatively and look for the good points in every person. Look and dig deep within... Every person was created by GOD and can do good. If we want to beat Amalek (within and perhaps outside) and reach world peace, health, and happiness in abundance for all, it is time to wake up and start respecting, accepting, loving, caring, teaching, and listening to our fellow brothers and sisters, no matter their background. A crucial lesson in the name of Rebbi Yitzchak of Berdichev, alav hashalom, is to be a Sanigor (a defender) of Beit Israel; protect them and speak well about them. As RAMAK (Rabbi Cordovero Alav Hashalom) said, if the Jew doesn't seem holy now, you must know his grandfather and forefathers were! So speak well about him/her!

Did someone hurt you? Consider this analogy. Say you are slicing some Muenster cheese, and you accidentally cut your finger. Would you take revenge by grabbing the knife and cutting your other hand? After all, it was your other hand that perpetrated the offense, was it not? Of course not.

Your other hand is as much a part of you as anything else. Revenge would be insane! When we learn to appreciate that we are all genuinely united, hurting the other guy by "paying him back" is as ridiculous as hurting yourself. In fact, if someone embarrasses or yells at you (wife, friends, work, etc.) and you stay quiet, you can reach the highest of all levels in your soul refinement.

That is why the Torah says, "Love your neighbor as yourself." If I realize that the other guy and I are part of the very same unit, then revenge is as silly as cutting my other hand with the knife. Similar phenomena have been recorded throughout time, as GOD must periodically resort to the most painful avenues to bring togetherness messages to the fore. How much healthier and more prudent would it be if only mankind learned this lesson on its own without the agonizing Divine intervention?

Parents naturally relate this way to their children. No matter how badly children misbehave, parents do not stop loving them. Annoyance? Yes. Reprimand? Of course. But normal parents do not take revenge on their children. They do not bear a grudge because they relate to their children as an extension of themselves; so, hurting our children is hurting ourselves. Since parents do not desire revenge, they can forget the bad things and focus on the good. That is why it is easy for parents to love their children.

This very same dynamic can work with any relationship! With parents and children, the process is more instinctive. But when it comes to marriage, the potential for oneness is even greater! Unlike the parent/child affiliation, spouses actually choose each other, allowing for the prospects for enhanced unity to be even greater! But it does take a lot more work...naturally. Please share this message. We are better than this; let's start working on our middot and open our hearts to love, respect, accept, support, and have each other's backs. This will increase joy and unity, and we will begin to love more and get closer every hour, every day, to the 3rd and final Beit Hamikdash.

We hope you take advantage of and apply for these lessons. In conclusion, it is important to note the Haftorah we read on Sukkot

(Zechariah) that speaks of the final Battle of Gog and Magog. If you feel stress or anxiety, take deep breaths to first relax your mind and slow down your heart rate. Focus on the stream of water that will flow from Jerusalem to Jericho. This heavenly blessed water will heal the sick and help grow medicinal plants and herbs in this vast, dry land.

There will be no more sickness in the world, and we will have a source of healing. Remember, GOD is capable of loving more in one second than we can ever love anyone in a lifetime. We cannot even comprehend His love for us. We are His children, His creation, and He is always ready to take us back with love and open arms. He is waiting for us to simply return to Him, and then He will crown this world with His Keter, and then the world will be a better place for our children and us.

13) Faith & Bitachon

Trusting in GOD and looking to Him alone creates a vessel with which to receive His blessing for all of one's needs. Then, when required, whatever one needs is sent (Likutai Maharani, 76), like the manna, "bread from Heaven." When a person puts all his trust in the Creator and realizes that he can achieve nothing without His help, the Creator will provide for his needs.

Whether it is health, sustenance, finding a spouse, raising children, or whatever you want to achieve, we must ask for assistance and trust in the Creator to provide. So even though we still have to work and put in a good measure of effort, we must learn the balance between trusting in GOD and doing our part.

What we acquire spiritually through trusting Hashem is brought into reality when we put in the required physical labor. Once we work on our faith, the next step is seeing it come alive. Then, the spiritual muscle of Emunah will flex into bitachon (higher confidence in our faith). Having bitachon gives us the ability to have confidence in our efforts and desires. The more faith you have, the less worry you have to carry on your shoulders!

Bitachon

More often than not, many of us experience moments in which life presents us with a situation where we find ourselves not in control. Unfortunately, we can do nothing to prevent the recurrence of such trying moments, and sometimes, this can even lead to despair. Therefore, it pays to work on our emunah muscles and build them up to more bitachon (so we never despair). This is because bitachon will fill in the significant gaps in a person's faith. Faith creates reality. For which we strive, and bitachon can reinforce our hold on it.

Tool

When you wake up in the morning, try to picture how you want your day to look, from the first step to the last. As you do this, remember that unexpected occurrences or pitfalls may occur, but your faith in GOD is the ladder you need to climb to reach your goal. You will find daily and weekly lessons and opportunities for self-growth.

This is the highest level of bitachon and faith that you understand everything that happens is for the best to learn and grow.

Another point for the Jewish sage in you is to learn a little Gemara in the morning, before you start your day, or in the evening, before you go to sleep. The three angels, Gavriel, Michael, and Raphael (G, M, R), are rooted in the word Gemara. Sages say they protect the ones who learn this when they leave their home or go to sleep.

Faith and bitachon (trust) are the foundation of the principal concerns of GOD's ways. Trusting in God creates a positive spiritual effect on a person. That is why the Creator creates various situations that allow a man to utilize his innate strengths in more practical and constructive ways. Let us never forget to thank the Creator for every success we experience!

14) Meditation for Mind and Soul (Recovery)

We highly recommend meditation as a way of reawakening or strengthening your spiritual and mental state. There are many meditation steps available in other books. Still, we find the three-step process created by the great sage and spiritual progenitor of Hasidic Jews, known as the Baal Shem Tov (literally, "Master of the Good Name").

Pat yourself on the back. At the same time, do not celebrate for too long! There is always more to learn and more to master. Remember, this book is not meant to transform you in a week or a month; we are talking about months and years, or maybe even longer. It depends on your work ethic and the teachers you surround yourself with.

Three-Step Process: Submit, Separate, Sweet.

Sweet Step 1: Submission

Meditate with deep breathing and speak to the Creator of the world. Yes, He is almighty, but He still listens to everyone who speaks to Him. Do a lot of deep breathing and imagine fresh air going to all areas of your body. Refresh and regenerate yourself with good thoughts and words. If you like music, put on some upbeat, uplifting music, or listen to the soothing sounds of nature.

Step 2: Separation

Learn to be aware and conscious of both your divine and animal souls: your yetzer hatov (divine) and yetzer hara (animalistic). It is imperative to understand which voice is your animal soul and which is coming from your divine soul. With time, you can master this and decipher them easily.

*As we have stated, we need both souls to advance and learn, but to become a master and a warrior in your own right, you must be able to separate them and unite them.

Step 3: Sweet

Once you attain clarity of mind, you will begin to understand things better. Once there, you are here; your thoughts and actions will be in sync. End your meditation with sweet words and a happy melody (known in Hasidic Jewish circles as a niggun).

You can also sing on your own from your heart.

SECTION IV

ESSENTIAL INSIGHTS

1) Hollywood and the Movies

It is very well known that movies are not what they used to be from decades past. Just ask your parents or grandparents. Once upon a time, a movie could provide meaning or historical references. Today, most of them look for ways to make the next big paycheck or lure you in many manipulative ways. We will let the research speak for itself, as numbers do not lie.

Researchers at Dartmouth Medical School in New Hampshire studied 6,500 American teens between the ages of 10 and 14 in a two-year study. The teens were regularly quizzed through confidential telephone surveys regarding how often and how much they were drinking, along with what potential influential factors factored into their decision-making.

The scientists, led by Dr. James Sargent, concluded that watching celebrities drink alcohol accounted for 28% of the proportion of teens who started drinking between surveys. In addition, 20% of those moved to binge drinking. Teens who watched movies that featured alcohol were 63% more likely to progress into binge drinking. The link was seen not just with the character drinking but also with alcohol placement in the films. Having friends who drink was the first influential factor, while movies were the third highest! Parents who drink and have the money to buy alcohol, and who can access drinks at home, were not ranked as the other risk factors. So, what can we take away from this?

Movies are real life for these people. They take the art of a movie and allow it to imitate their life, thinking that movies reflect the real world, where everyone is doing just the same. The same concept applies to drugs, violence, etc. But unfortunately, it becomes the norm after a while, and people become desensitized.

As a parent or teacher, it is essential to educate our children with facts and to become more media savvy in understanding the world of movies or television. Many celebrities or athletes have a tragic ending to their lives, so it is important to share an open dialogue with kids. We must make our children feel comfortable and share information with us; take an interest in them. Otherwise, if our children feel like they cannot share things with us, they will go out and act on these deviant behaviors.

Before I wrote this book, I was also involved in athletics and enjoyed watching many movies until I was educated on their effects. I am sure there are positive films out there, but the more you understand, the more you will see how superficial it all is and how much they hurt us more than they help. Realize how valuable time is and how you do not want to waste it. Here, you will see how the Samech Mem, the evil husks/forces of this world, feed off negative movies and more. So, spend time working on yourself and your loved ones and/or your community. Then, create your own movie, become your star, search for the truth, and be the best person you can become; it will pay off better than any movie out there!

2) Internet Realities

It is not just in the Orthodox communities, but worldwide, that the Internet has not become a safe place. The Gedolai Hador (the greatest leader of the Jewish people) warned us against the threats and manipulations of the internet many years ago. We will let the numbers and research speak to you, and you will see how accurate the results appear.

The online world opens the door for trusting young people to interact with virtual strangers, even people they would usually cross the street to avoid in real life. But, unfortunately, about 1 in 7 kids have been sexually solicited online, says John Shehan, CyberTipline program manager for the National Center for Missing and Exploited Children in Alexandria, Virginia. CyberTipline helps prevent sexual exploitation of children by reporting cases of kids enticed online to do sexual acts.

Shehan also mentions, "While sexual predators have targeted children in chat rooms, they migrate to wherever young people go online. More predators are now scouring social networking sites because these sites have centralized so much information." A child's profile typically includes photos, personal interests, and blogs.

He adds, "In terms of predators, that is a hot spot where they can go to research victims; they need to meet these kids, groom these children, and become friends." Predators may take on fake identities and feign interest in a child's favorite bands, TV shows, video games, or hobbies. These online trolls may approach the child as a newbie.

Acquired a best friend. They will make it seem like they have much in common, "similar likes and dislikes. It is quite crafty what these child predators will go through."

Internet Safety Tips:

Some tips from Netsmartz.org for responding to cyberbullying:

- Experts say that kids should never share Internet passwords with anyone other than parents to keep others from using their email and Internet accounts.
- If children are harassed or bullied through instant messaging, help them use the "block" or "ban" feature to prevent the bully from contacting them.
- If a child keeps getting harassing emails, delete that email account (after saving copies of the messages) and set up a new one. Remind your child to give the new email address only to family and a few trusted friends.

Tell your child not to respond to rude or harassing emails, messages, or postings. If the cyberbullying continues, call the police. Keep a record of the emails as proof. Ask your children if they use a social networking site. Look at the site together or search for it yourself online. Social networking sites often have age limits. Tell your kids not to post a full name, address, phone number, school name, or other personal information to help a stranger find them.

Remind them that photos, like your child in a team sweatshirt, can give away clues about where they live. Ask them not to send photos to people they meet online. Learn about privacy settings that allow kids to choose who can view their profiles. Explain that strangers who approach them online are not always who they say they are and that it is dangerous to meet them in real life. Tell them to "instant message" only with family or friends, whom they already know offline.

When it comes to Internet safety, there is no substitute for parental supervision. Put your computer in a common area of your home, not a child's bedroom, so that you can keep an eye on online activities. Go to websites that explain the shorthand kids use in instant messaging, like "POS" ("parent over shoulder") or "LMIRL" ("let's meet in real life"), so you know what is going on.

Ask your kids to report any online sexual solicitation to you or another trusted adult right away. Shehan asks adults to report the event to the CyberTipline (8008435678), where staff will contact law enforcement agencies to investigate. He also advises parents to call their local police and save all offensive emails as evidence.

Internet Danger #3: Pornography

One of the worst dangers of the Internet, for many parents, is the idea that pornography could pop up and surprise their children. However, parents may not realize that some kids are actually going online to seek out web porn.

As advised by John Shehan, you can view the Internet browser history to see which websites your child may be visiting. Nonetheless, tech-savvy young teens can delete their history, and so you must install internet filtering software to block porn sites in the first place.

Internet safety tips

- Install Internet filtering software to block porn sites from any computer or phone your child has access to. Use filtering software that monitors and records instant messaging and chat room conversations and websites visited. Use a monitoring program that filters pornography keywords in several languages. Why? Some teens have figured out how to get around filters by typing in porn-related search terms in other languages.

Internet Danger #4: Damaged Reputations

Camera phones, digital cameras, and webcams are everywhere these days, and kids can be victims of their own inexperience with new technology.

Many post pictures, videos, or notes online that they later regret. John Shehan also advises, "Think before you post, because once you do, it is going to be up there forever."

A child's online reputation is a growing concern, Aftab says, with the rise of online social networking and profiles. She cites reports of

Schools and employers reject young people for high school programs, internships, college admissions, and jobs after reviewing what applicants have posted online.

Many teenage girls put up provocative photos of themselves, Shehan says. Why? Handy, a teenager herself, believes it is a game of one-upmanship. "Kids are trying to look cool. They're doing it because everyone else is doing it. So, a girl will see a picture and say, 'Oh, I can top that.' And before you know it, she's half naked on the Internet for everybody to see."

Internet safety tips

- Explain that others may have already copied them into public forums and websites, even if your kids delete their posted photos.
- Tell your kids not to let anyone, even friends, take pictures or videos of them that could cause embarrassment online, such as if a relative or teacher saw them.
- Talk to your kids about possible consequences, the experts say. For example, a 17-year-old might think it is hilarious to post a photo of himself looking drunk, with empty beer bottles strewn around him. But will a college admissions officer be impressed? Probably not.

Cell Phones

According to the British Chiropractic Association, our obsession with smartphones has led to a rise in young people with back pain.

Problems. The amount of time spent leaning over small phone screens can put spinal discs under pressure. Thanks to our technological lifestyle, 45 percent of 16- to 24-year-olds suffer from back pain—a 60 percent rise from last year. Aching backs are not the only unhealthy consequence of your mobile phone. Here are why smartphones are bad for your physical, mental, and emotional health.

Accidents

If you are looking at your phone, then you are more likely to walk into a lamppost, trip over your feet, or have a more severe accident. Carnegie Mellon University researchers have found that drivers listening to someone talk on their mobile devices have a 37% reduction in brain activity. Meanwhile, a University of Washington study found that texting pedestrians were four times more likely to ignore the lights or forget to look for traffic before crossing.

Anxiety

Instead of making us more connected, the potential for continuous smartphone communication can make us feel more isolated. Young adults who spend 11 hours looking at their screens every day expect constant updates from their friends, and a lull in messages can lead to anxiety. Dr. Richard Graham, a psychologist specializing in technology addiction at Nightingale Hospital, states, "There's a terrible feeling that the person is ignoring you; young people have to manage to feel excluded by people who are very.

important to them."

Obesity

Consultant orthopedic surgeon Jonathan Dearing, spokesman for the Royal College of Surgeons of Edinburgh, says that the technology revolution has led to "reduced physical activity and obesity," the fourth most significant cause of death worldwide. Dearing mentions, "If someone is on the floor above you at work, rather than going to see them, you will send an email. You would phone up a friend rather than travel to meet them; inactivity leads to obesity, which means the risk of cardiovascular disease is greatly increased. Pretty much every pathology—such as breast cancer, prostate cancer, or bowel cancer—you are both more likely to get and less likely to recover from if you are inactive."

Depression

Child psychotherapist Julie Lynn Evans spoke on how she dealt with one or two attempted suicides a year in the 1990s but now faces up to four a month. Lynn Evans blames smartphones for this increase, saying that "it allows teenagers to carry a world of cyberbullying with them wherever they go. There are difficult chat rooms, self-harming websites, anorexia websites, pornography, and a whole invisible world of dark places. In real life, we travel with our children. When they are connected via their smartphone to the web,

They usually travel alone."

Sleeping with the phone?

More than 60% of 18- to 29-year-old smartphone users take their phones to bed. Nonetheless, studies have found that just two hours of exposure to brightly lit screens can suppress melatonin and lead to sleeping troubles. Professor Kevin Morgan, Director of the Clinical Sleep Research Unit at Loughborough University, mentions how late-night intellectual stimulation from our phones makes it more difficult to relax. But, Professor Morgan explains, "Why are you looking at a screen before you go to bed? It could be because you are working. Or a child might be playing an exciting game. Looking at screens engages you in intellectual activity in a way that is not like reading a book. It puts you in a state of alertness, which is the last thing you want to be before going to bed."

Relationships

Social skills have also depleted, thanks to focusing on our smartphones instead of those around us. This is particularly obvious among children, who are increasingly ignored by wise, phone-obsessed parents. Jenny Radesky, a pediatrician specializing in child development, shares with us that "children learn by watching us how to have a conversation and how to read other people's facial expressions. If that is not happening, children are missing out on important development milestones."

Attention span

You are much less likely to finish reading this book if you are on your mobile device when you have the option of clicking to see a heartbreaking video of a child with his pet or your friends' photos. Research has found that smartphones significantly reduce our attention spans and make us far less effective at completing difficult and detailed tasks. Even the mere presence of a smartphone is distracting enough to ruin our mental concentration.

Solutions and Tips:

Educate others on the risks of the internet and smartphones. Understand that you are literally feeding or sustaining the evil forces of this world by giving power to the negative aspects of movies and the internet.

Instead, be a hero; support the positive energies.

One is allowed and should use the internet for work and/or cooking, banking, legal, shopping, and other essential tasks. Understand how to go about it and educate yourself to protect yourself, your family, and the direction of the world. Yes, with every click, you can affect the world; that is how powerful each human is once you share Torah classes or guide others.

We recommend installing a filter on all your computers and smartphones, and maybe even consider purchasing a phone with no camera.

Internet. If not, go with filtered phones. Just like you would get any regular filter (like McAfee and others), why not get something more robust with more support for today's growing needs?

I am sure there are other people out there helping, but a few filter groups recommend, and I have dealt with:

https://tag.org/ is a community service for computers, smartphones, laptops, tablets, and other digital devices to be filtered to prevent access to inappropriate material, etc. These are also two direct filtering companies:

https://gentechsolution.com/

https://www.techloq.com/# Contact us.

When it comes to raising kids or teaching the youth, yes, filters can help, but the internet at home and on phones is a challenge. We are all facing an actual test of controlling one's desires and inclinations for the greater good. Check here for inspiration: https://theprojectfocus.org/inspiration/

A filter is a must in today's society; we advise you to contact https://tag.org/. With physical locations in many major cities all over the world. Phone: 7327301824   Email: tag@tag.org. Along with methodology, we advise heartfelt prayers and seeking the wisdom of God-fearing rabbis in your community.

3) Shalom Bayit and Chinuch (Parenting)

First things first, I am in no position to educate other parents, as I am still learning. Therefore, I will humbly share what I have learned and simply pass it along. Firstly, I will give credit to the greats and to those I am still learning from. Before we get to parenting, the number 1 thing is Shalom Bayit. Below is a Shiur every single married man must listen to and apply to this life daily:

https://613tube.com/watch/?v=QBGN2N6Wro4

He brings sources from Chessed Le Avraham, Hida, Pele Yoetz, and more, on the way to "gauge" how your avodat Hashem is. How are you serving Hashem? In Shamyim, they check his home! They check his wife. So if your wife doesn't do what you want? How do you react? Our reactions with our wife and kids are the trust test. If your service of Hashem is good, then your wife will treat you well. A man must never scream or be angry at his wife. He should smile and be as happy as he can at home. Take the hits like a man, stay calm and quiet, and be happy (hard to do), but with time you serve Hashem, and correct things will be good at home.

If you follow this, you won't need these marriage counselors or therapists; take care of your home, and Hashem will take care of the rest. In shul, kollel, and outside, he can be as serious and strict as he wants. Don't judge your wife negatively; no matter if she is on the phone or not, be modest at the moment. Pretend you don't see it. Work on improving your relationship with Hashem. Your wife or daughter

Cannot rebuke well; girls are different from boys. See the long-term goal. Let the small things go; it will get better; listen to the Rabbi's advice in the lecture above. At home, a different hat must be worn, one full of patience, mercy, love, and happiness. Listen to class; he says if you need to rebuke your wife, then do it, that you must change, or in the 3rd person, or say it's your fault—maybe you did this in the past! A woman is not built in her nature to hear rebuke well from her husband. Our job is to teach lovingly and keep them happy. If she is upset at you, never answer or respond; this will remove past sins. Try to always say yes, sweetheart, honey, etc. These are secrets to a happy home. Once you have mastered this, the rest will more or less fall in place; we have included more info to help.

With parenting and educating the youth, more attention needs to be put in place. Many of today's rabbis and scholars print books solely on this topic of educating children on what we call Chinuch (Jewish Education).

Perhaps Judaism's most vital institution and role in existence is the next generation's education. So many people did not grow up with a father or mother, but the points we will go through can be really beneficial for any teacher to learn and provide these tools to their students or parents themselves.

In addition, the three books below are what I highly recommend to any educator and/or parent:

1. Planting & Building in Education: Raising a Jewish Child by Rabbi Shlomo Wolbe

2. Spare The Child by Rabbi Yechiel Yaakovson

3. On His Path by Rabbi Shlomo Goldberg

It is essential to realize that not everyone has the privilege of having both a mother and a father. So, if your parents are still around, please stop right now and call them and give them your thanks for partnering with GOD to bring you to this world and give you the gift of life. If your parents are not around, pray to them and thank them, or perhaps learn about doing a kaddish for them (ask your local Orthodox rabbi). Now, if you are an educator or a parent, please embrace this role and learn as much as you can to help other parents out there; they are doing the best they can in building the future leaders of this world.

With my little experience, I can share what I have learned: that each parent's role is unique. I was in a lecture from an expert educator, Rabbi Shlomo Goldberg, and below is what I learned. Just like GOD, first built a blueprint/plan for the creation of the world. So, must parents create a plan for their creation of this world? This will require further education beyond this book, but I can give you a small head start. Just like in sports, each player must know their role and responsibilities. For instance, a mother has a role that she can do better than the father, and vice versa. Well, some super moms can do both, but of course, to keep a healthy balance and not to get burned out, you need to understand both roles.

A mother is the one who has the power to build or break a home. She molds all the pieces and resources, while the father offers and

Created with them. She is the vessel that holds the "water," or the blessings of the Father.

She is the ultimate warrior who has the skills to cook, clean, and whip the children into shape. But, most importantly, the mom has a unique role in creating trust with her children. No matter what the child goes through, the safety and trust of a mom and child will feel safe. For instance, I heard a story of a three-year-old child who broke his arm and had to get a cast put on. He was in the most painful stages of the procedure when his mom stepped in and took a long, in-depth look into his eyes and told him, "Everything is going to be alright." The child stopped crying. He was calm and in a completely different state of mind. The doctor was shocked and said some teens, maybe even adults, cannot shift their focus like that. Well, yes, that is the power of a mom that builds trust in her children. Of course, there is plenty more on this, but this is not a book on chinuch. We advise you to learn more on your own.

A father has two unique roles: a leader and a friend. Especially with the challenges we face today, a father must lead his home with the utmost safety. He must be strong and create a "submarine" of his home that nobody can break into. He must create a strong and safe place for his family. Kids must feel, at most, that their home is the safest place: physically, emotionally, and spiritually. The key is to allow the kids to feel that they can tell Dad anything, just like a best friend.

This is harder said than done; discipline is involved, but of course, this requires more education and more in-depth learning. A short point:

when it comes to discipline, both parents need to take on this role. Nonetheless, the role should be similar to how GOD disciplines us in His concept of "Nase VeNIshma," meaning, "We will do, and we will listen." It is also important to have your kids do what you tell them and then explain the reasons afterward. To build up to this, try to compliment your child properly and give them plenty of encouragement. Make it real and make it count. The keywords for parenting are the big three: firm, fair, and friendly.

Transitions are a great time to build bonds with children. For instance, when kids wake up or come home from school, it can be scary. They must have a haven or a comfort zone to lean back on. Provide them with smiles and good feelings during these transitions. Parents or teachers can lead not only by voice and techniques but also by behavior. Perhaps some say the most important thing a parent or teacher can do is to lead by example. Yes, this implies being the person you want your kids to be. You cannot teach them about GOD if you are breaking GOD's rules yourself. You must remember that kids are always watching. So, think twice about what you wear or how you eat or talk; they watch and listen. If you want your kids or students to change, then you must be that change.

Here is a good audio class for men only to initiate the change, and their wives and households will follow if done properly. The Man's Enlightening the Wife—FOR MEN ONLY. MP3 https://on.soundcloud.com/nYco4PwQG22P6aK6iX

Safeguarding Intimate Forces

Intimate relations, if indulged in, can be like junk food. Sexual temptations come finely packaged but are bound to leave us feeling sick and disgusted with ourselves and with our partners, too. So how do you improve this diet? First, you go for more natural, wholesome "foods." By this, I mean an intimate relationship. Just like eating healthier, more natural, whole foods makes you feel better, so will a wholesome relationship.

This refers to being intimate with only one marriage partner. Discussing below will help us better understand the forces connected with sexuality, which are genuinely double-edged. When they are separated from their real purpose, they can push people to terrible forms of degradation. The purpose of the sexual act is to create life and the creation and strengthening of the relationship. When it is indulged purely for the sake of gratification, it betrays a callous disregard for the preciousness of life.

People who act this way may give the outward appearance of seeking closeness to a partner. But in reality, they are looking for a situation in which their desires will be gratified.

The Remedy for Lustful Forces

1. Strengthen our awareness that GOD, in His love and strength, is always close by to release us from the pressures and troubles that may surround us, even when a person becomes overwhelmed by the temptation to choose evil. GOD's desire is not to punish but to enable us to have power over our thoughts, minds, and bodies. Try having a conversation with GOD when you are stuck in traffic, before you go to bed, after a workout, or at any time. Give thanks and ask GOD for clarity (this can bring about amazing miracles at the right time).

2. Confession in words is necessary because man is primarily a creature of language. Whatever we may want to say about life and its situations expresses our entire system of belief and outlook. We may speak in a way that brings out how all of life, with all its details, is a quest to reveal godliness. On the simplest level, the cup is either half-full or half-empty.

3. If we are to lead our lives as we should, we must put our ideas, thoughts, words, and actions in order. We must know the truth of our existence and our condition, and that GOD has sent everything into our lives. So even when things are dark, and we seem to be encompassed by confusion, frustration, obstacles, or threats, GOD is with us. It is He who has sent the situation and He who will assist us in drawing us out of it. The three points above are excerpts from Rabbi Nachman's Tikkun (compiled and translated by Avraham Greenbaum).

When we keep these points in mind and abide by them, we find ourselves growing in our relationship with the Creator. It will also lead us to wholesome relationships that result in beautiful marriages. To get a better sense of why sexual forces were instituted and how they got there, we need to delve into the secrets of the Torah. With the help of our generation's great Rabbis, we were able to see that the Zohar (Kedoshim, p. 83, with the explanation of R. Daniel Frisch in his Matok Midvash) To get clarity on these, we need to date back to the first incident of sexuality with Adam and Eve (more in the Soul section).

The Zohar tells us that when Adam was first created, he did not benefit from the physical world since his very body/being was entirely spiritual. For instance, "When the body of Adam came to the world, the sun and the moon of this world saw him, and their lights were obscured before his, just like the light of a candle in the daylight... When Adam sinned by eating from the Tree of Knowledge, this caused a blemish in all the worlds, and they all descended from their previous levels." The supernal light that had previously shone upon him was darkened. He required a new body made of physical flesh and skin from this world, as it says, "And the Lord GOD made for Adam and his wife garments of skin and clothed them" (Genesis 3:21).

This was their physical body that could benefit from the bodily lusts of the physical world. To further understand this, we take a piece from the great Rav Shalom Arush's Shalita book, The Garden.

Of Peace, translated by a man of great inspiration to me, Rav Lazer Brody Shalita.

Only after the sin of the Tree of Knowledge were Adam and Eve clothed in garments of skin, physical bodies that could benefit from the physical lusts of this world. The experience of sexual lust came about as a punishment for the physical darkness forced upon Adam because of his sin. Before his sin, his body was entirely pure and shone brighter than the sun and the moon. Until then, his bonding with Eve took place on a wholly spiritual level and was utterly removed from lust and physical pleasure.

A wife's happiness and peace in the home depend entirely on the husband's holiness. This holiness is twofold, referring to the day-to-day conduct of the husband with his wife; in other words, he should treat her with love and respect. Second, his conduct with her during their days of the union should also be loving, characterized by kindness and consideration for her needs, rather than by his animal lusts.

The basic level is the husband's adherence to the religious law, halacha, in all aspects of marital relations. The highly regarded Rabbi Nachman of Breslov said:

"When my days have ended, and I leave this world, I will intercede for anyone who comes to my grave, recite these ten psalms, and give charity. No matter how grave his sins and transgressions are, I will do everything in my power to save him and cleanse him; I will span the length and breadth of the creation for them. I will take hold of his peyote (side curls) and pull him out of

Gehinnom!"

"I am very positive about everything I say. But I am more positive about this than about anything when I say that these Psalms help very, very much. These are the ten psalms: 16, 32, 41, 42, 59, 77, 90, 105, 137, and 150."

These psalms make up his Tikkun Haklali (General Remedy); it has many far-reaching benefits, as they have the power to remedy all kinds of negative thoughts and feelings. The ten psalms correspond to the ten archetypal types of the song, which vitalize the ten primary "pulses" governing the energy system of the human soul and body.

Though it was initially revealed as a remedy for the damage caused by the wasteful emission of the seed by males, the recital of the Tikkun HaKlali applies to men and women alike. More can be read about this ISH PELE (man of wonders/miracles) here: https://breslov.org/. Perhaps the most powerful teaching that has to do with guarding the covenant (brit) is contained in Rabbi Nachman's teaching. He also talks beautifully about AZAMRA (finding good points in each other). If we can fix the Ahavat Israel and the covenant, we are in amazing shape to bring the redemption ASAP. His teaching contains all you need to know, and his teaching will be a blaze (fire) to help us till Mashiach comes; not enough can be said about how hard he worked to help this last generation!

Angels Today

What does Judaism say about angels? Are they involved in our lives? I have always felt like I have a guardian angel, but I would like to know more. Does it have a name? How do I communicate with it?

The Aish Rabbi Replies:

First, let's try to understand exactly what an angel is. If you see little children flying around your head with their wings flapping happily behind them, do not think these are angels. They are hallucinations! Real angels do not have bodies, wings, or one drop of physicality. They are often described as winged humans (Exodus 25:17, Isaiah 6:2, Ezekiel 1:5, and 10:18) to help us understand their essence. This is similar to how the Torah describes GOD as having a "strong hand and outstretched arm." Of course, GOD does not have an arm! Instead, the Torah conveys to us something about GOD's mighty strength in a way that we can understand. (Maimonides—Book of Knowledge 2:4)

Angels are defined as metaphysical beings who are messengers of GOD. They are spiritual, but they have no free will. They can only do precisely what they have been commanded to do by their Creator.

The word "Malach" (Hebrew for angel) means messenger, which also translates as work. So, in other words, an angel is a "messenger" of GOD who carries out His work. Similarly, the English word "angel" comes from the Greek word "Angelos," meaning "messenger" or "agent."

Angels are sometimes referred to as the "Heavenly Court" because they administer the work of the King, GOD. That is to say, just as a king makes plans but his court discharges them, so too God makes plans, and His angels discharge them.

This is the meaning of the Midrash, which says, "No blade of grass grows without an angel telling it to 'Grow!'" This teaches us that everything on earth has a spiritual counterpart that influences it. Even a blade of grass has an angel looking over it to ensure it receives nourishment or causes it to die at its appointed time. Nations also have angels assigned to them.

For example, the Torah recounts the famous story of Jacob fighting with Samael, the angel of Esav. (See Genesis 32:5, Midrash Genesis Rabbah 10:6, and "The Way of GOD" 2:5:3.) Each angel has only one particular task to fulfill.

The most well-known angels are

- Micha'el (literally, "Who is like GOD") carries out GOD's kindness missions. First, he accompanies a person on the right side since "right" is always associated with kindness.
- Gavriel ("My strength is GOD") is on the left side, which is
- always associated with the attributes of strength and judgment.
- Uriel ("My light is GOD") goes in front of a person as if illuminating the proper path to go.
- Raphael ("My healer is GOD") protects a person from harm and goes behind a person to "cover the backside."

Interestingly, we find three of these angels visiting Abraham in Genesis 18:2. Micha'el (kindness) had come to bring Sarah the good news of her pregnancy, Gavriel (judgment) came to overthrow Sodom, and Raphael (healing) came to heal Abraham following his circumcision. The angels, such as those who spoke to Abraham, were purely spiritual forces of inhuman form.

Due to their unique nature, it is impossible to communicate with angels, although there have been stories of great sages who could do so.

It is certainly forbidden to pray to angels. Not only is it forbidden, but it would be a waste of time since angels can only do what GOD tells them
 them to do anyway!

However, GOD always has an attentive ear to his children, and He is waiting for your prayers. Reading the bedtime Shema, a beautiful prayer about the four protecting angels mentioned above, is one good place to start.

When you perform a mitzvah, you create an angel that accompanies you. The commandments that form that attachment are the true "guardian angels" of a person.

4) The Comeback/Return

In my youth, I did some horrible things—both unethical and illegal. Is it possible to make amends for having lived a sinful lifestyle? Sometimes I feel so low that I cannot imagine how I will ever get back up. Is my soul permanently stained by all this?

The Aish Rabbi Replies:

It is never too late. As Rabbi Yisrael Salanter was known to say, "As long as the flame is burning, we can still make amends."

Teshuva is the Jewish idea of return. When we do teshuva, we examine our ways, identify those areas where we are losing ground, and return to our previous state of spiritual purity. In the process, we are returning to our connection with the Almighty as well.

Teshuva was created even before the world was created because GOD knew that it would be needed. Nothing stands in the way of teshuva, and the very fact that you have made the critical step of writing this letter means that you have already begun the process of teshuva. We must try to always be in a constant state of teshuva.

For successful teshuva, we have to realize that GOD loves us even in light of all the mistakes we have made. Realize that GOD understands you, that He is "cheering you on," and wants to help. Do not feel guilty; any mistakes you have made are part of a growth process to get where you are today.

Growth is what GOD created us for, and even hardships are the best thing for us. GOD is not the "big bully in the sky"; He is on your side. The Talmud states that if you do teshuva out of love, you can even transform your mistakes into mitzvahs (Yoma 86b). Sort of like "dry cleaning for the soul."

The process of Teshuva involves these steps, which we have derived from halachayomit.com and the teachings of the Torah giant Harav Ovadia Yosef, who has left this world, but his teachings and books are thriving so much in so many of our daily lives.

Step 1 – The Mitzvah of Confession

Verbally, articulate the mistake and ask for forgiveness.

Regret. Realizing the extent of the damage and feeling sincere regret.

Step 2 – Commitment to the Future

Cessation. Immediately stopping the harmful action.

Step 3 – Remorse

Truly feeling remorse for the sin in one's heart. Finally, resolving. Making a firm commitment not to repeat it in the future.
However, these steps go only so far. If our past actions have hurt another, we must ask for their forgiveness.

The Mitzvah of Confession

The Rambam writes (at the beginning of his Hilchot Teshuva) that if one transgresses any of the Torah's commandments either knowingly or unknowingly, when one repents, one must confess one's sin before Hashem, as the verse states, "If a man or woman performs any sin, etc., unknowingly, confess the sin which they have committed," which refers to actually confessing one's sin verbally.

This confession is a positive Torah commandment.

How should one confess? One must say, "Please, Hashem, I have sinned, transgressed, and committed iniquities before you, and I now regret and am ashamed of my actions, and I shall never again do this" (meaning that one must accept upon himself never to commit this sin again). This is the primary aspect of the confession. The more one confesses and speaks lengthily in this manner, the more praiseworthy one is. This was indeed the practice when the Beit Hamikdash stood, when a sinner would bring a "Chatat" or "Asham" offering to atone for his sin, he would confess his sin upon the offering, for if one does not repent for one's sin, one will not achieve atonement even if one brings one thousand offerings to Hashem. Thus, confession is an integral part of the Teshuva process, and one who has not confessed his sin has not fulfilled the Mitzvah of Teshuva.

Nowadays, when the Beit Hamikdash, unfortunately, lies in ruins and we have no Mizbeach (altar) to offer our sacrifices on, all we
I have left Teshuva. Indeed, one who repents fully shall not be reminded at all of one's sins on the Day of Reckoning.

Commitment to the Future

Another provision of the mitzvah of Teshuva is that the repentant individual must accept upon himself never to return to his sin again. For instance, if one transgresses a negative Torah commandment, such as Shabbat desecration, or if one eats foods requiring checking for worms without checking, one must wholeheartedly accept never again. Repeating the sin. Similarly, suppose one has transgressed a positive Torah commandment, such as not reciting Kiddush on Shabbat or not honoring one's parents adequately. In that case, one must accept to perform these mitzvot properly. However, if one says, "I shall sin, and I shall repent," he will never be allowed to repent.

Remorse

Likewise, one must feel remorse for the sins one has committed by realizing the wickedness of one's actions and how much it has angered his Creator. However, if one does not regret one's deeds, even if one forsakes the sin completely and never performs it again, and even if one has confessed one's sin, one has not fulfilled the mitzvah of Teshuva. Therefore, one will remain unforgiven for his sin.

Based on the above, there are three primary aspects of Teshuva: verbally confessing one's sin, accepting oneself never again to commit these sins, and genuinely feeling remorse for the sin in one's heart. If one does all of these things, one has fulfilled the Mitzvah of Teshuva is beloved by his Creator. Rabbi Akiva once exclaimed,

"Fortunate are you, Israel!

Before Whom are you becoming purified, and Who is purifying you? Your Father in Heaven! As the verse states, "The mikveh (hope) of Israel is Hashem—just as a mikveh purifies the impure, so does Hashem purify the Jewish nation."

5) Time management

The average life span is 25,000 days, or roughly seventy years, with some fortunate enough to live 35,000 days, or close to ninety years.

There are still many people who live for as long as eighty years, approximately 28,835 days. The following average subdivision of regular activities during one twenty-four-hour period comes from

Rabbi Chanan Gordon, who, through his list, helps us better understand what our lives are made of in terms of time:

We, in the modern Western nations, spend on average:

18,477 days sleeping.

1,635 days of eating.

3,202 days working.

1,999 days commuting to work and home.

2,676 days in recreation/entertainment.

1,576 days of shopping.

720 days in community activities.

671 days in the bathroom.

576 days caring for the needy and other acts of kindness.

The precious time left over from the above list is a mere 7,336 days. This means we have a little more than seven thousand days in which to make a difference in our lives and the lives of others. You can easily see how utterly important getting a handle on time management truly is. We need to make time management a priority in our lives to get into the Garden, also known as Olam Haba, literally "the next world," or, as it is commonly referred to, the world to come.

The Miracle of the Bamboo Tree and Patience

Consider a different dream, a dream of a simple farmer. It is the story of a sort of five-year plan that belongs to the Creator of Everything! Yet, the dream is the same as every farmer willing to learn perhaps the most significant lesson the Creator has given the human race: patience. There once lived a simple Chinese man who had a simple dream. And he prayed for the fulfillment of this dream, night and day: he prayed to the Creator of the universe, to a Higher Power, to help him feed his family.

One day, the farmer, who desperately wanted to feed and clothe his family, heard talk among other farmers about this nearly "magical seed" from which would sprout a legendary tree. All one had to do was plant it and nurture it. Becoming excited, believing this to be an answer to his prayers. One of his great Chinese sages would have called it the "will of Heaven." The farmer got one of these seeds and rushed to his languishing farm to make preparations for planting, and Heaven is praised for eventual harvesting.

When the day of planting came, and with visions of a thankfully sated family before his eyes, he ceremonially dug the plot for the first seed and gratefully dropped it into the hole. This ageless story of hope and despair, followed by more hope, continues. Day after day, the farmer dutifully hauled buckets of water to water the seed, and no small feat it was, for he had to travel a great distance to fetch the water from the nearest source.

The first year of planting is not a spring, not a shoot, and has absolutely no evidence of any growth whatsoever. The farmer despaired in the second year; nothing, only the farmer's despair, was watered by his tears. In the third season, no plant emerged from the well-watered seed. In the fourth season, the only thing looming before the hardworking farmer was a mountain of anguish and heartache, as he realized that he might have been deceived by the promises of this "God-given seed," and he went home to face the many questions from his increasingly hungry family, who barely subsisted on the small yield from his other crops during all those years of waiting.

The fifth year arrived, only to see a now-defeated farmer making one last journey to take one last haul of water to the spot to ensure that it was adequately watered. Nothing. But then, just a few days later, the farmer saw something creeping up from the plot of land.

He could see not only evidence of growth, but right before his eyes, just over a few months, the bamboo tree reached the majestic heights of the farmer's dreams. First, ten feet, twenty feet, thirty, and forty, at last, to the laughs and amazement of the farmer, of his truly grateful and expectant family, and of all his curious neighbors, who had been scoffing at his attempts and goading him to give up hope. The bamboo, which after five years of painstakingly careful nurturing, finally burst forth like a spacecraft hurtling toward a new horizon, ultimately reached ninety feet!

Such is GOD's "five-year plan"—such a simple yet powerful testimony that the Creator of the universe loves and nurtures the hopes and dreams of humanity. In return, the least we can show is the love of one's fellow neighbor, as shown in acts of kindness and patience. Hashem wants His creatures to practice and nurture patience.

6) Responsibility on Earth

Some of you might say we do not care for these pro athletes or Hollywood stars. One might say I am nothing like them. We have a responsibility on this Earth. Especially the ones who are part of the chosen nation must speak up and educate ourselves and our communities, and then the rest of the world will, God willing. follow.

As we said, many of our youth and children are watching today's Hollywood and sports. It is quite an apparent look at what is going on in the world news. What was once important—faith, family, and doing things for the greater good—seems to have slowly diminished in the growing superficial areas of commercials, money, fashion, and sports. Marketing in today's society can negatively affect values.

We teach children. Society's values are changing, and if we do not build awareness and boundaries, it can damage the people we love most.

It is not what it used to be; it is just better to accept the world is changing and ask how we can adapt and prepare for the next. Generation.

Preparing the next generation of children (whether it is parenting or teaching), we need to understand that many of these kids may end up watching these players on TV and the internet and will likely want to follow their careers/lives. Therefore, it is essential to prepare and educate our youth as best as possible.

We must be interested as parents, teachers, or community members to educate and address concerns. We must reemphasize that kids are innocent and often not at fault; they do things based on what the world feeds them without the proper filter. This is why kids are bound to get into trouble in today's society. However, many of them cannot blame what today's media and the internet are showing them.

Well, here is some good news. There is still plenty of good in this world, and we can tap into some of it. It is never too late, and we must focus on not only the good but the truth as well (or, in Hebrew, the Emet). The world stands on goodness, lovingkindness, judgment, justice, and truth.

7) The Huddle

Growing up, I remember watching many teams in huddles (basketball, baseball, or football). A huddle is special. It can turn the game around and put things into perspective. It is what I call an energy field of unity that combines a group into one unit.

Some can further describe it as a quick adjustment in the game, but many with a more profound sense of the game's art know there is something deeper behind it. It is a connection you get with others that puts you back into rhythm.

Many times, athletes pray or coach themselves. What are they doing? How does it help? When in the middle of a game or life and getting out of touch, we need to take a break or find a way to get back into focus. Many of us do this differently; this source is an essential tool to help get us in touch with our inner self, or what many call our soul or spirit. In the next section, we will clarify the pressures we face in the game and in life.

We do not always have a team or huddle to help us focus, so we need to take a few deep breaths to get our minds back on focusing. How can we battle and better understand setbacks and challenges? Where does it come from, and how can we shift our mindset to be prepared for those challenges? We will attempt to answer these questions with the help of Coach Y.

Coach Y

Below is an intense yet powerful letter from GYE (Guard Your Yes), a platform by Rabbi Dr. Abraham J. Twerski, a psychologist and master scholar. He gives a unique view of the Yetzer Hara (evil inclination) and how we view it mentally as a coach. I.e., someone who gives us a hard time but does this to make us better, push us to our limits, and see how far and great the human being can become when pushed correctly. Below is the letter used in the allegory with a boxing coach, which perfectly explains our "training" approach to this world.

8) A Letter from the Yetzer Hara

To my star pupil, I am writing this letter to let you know what I think of you. Up here in Heaven, things are not like they are down on Earth. Over there, people only know what they can see. If they see a person as "successful," they think that he is the greatest guy. When they see somebody struggling, they think he might be one of the weaker elements.

Let me tell you something. Hashem gives every person a certain ability that nobody knows about, down where you live. Some people are capable of tremendous things, while others are put there for much smaller purposes. In His infinite wisdom, only Hashem can give every person exactly what he needs to reach his potential. I am very misunderstood. Most people hate me, and I don't blame them. Most people think that my job is to make sure that they fail in all aspects of Mitzvos and that I rejoice every time they sin. This is the furthest thing from the truth. Did you ever watch a boxing coach train his students? It is a funny sight.

The coach will put on gloves and fight against his students. Initially, he won't strike him or throw his best punches. But as the student gets better and better, the coach will fight him harder and harder. He does this to improve his skills and become the best boxer he can be. This is where it gets strange. Every time the coach knocks down the student, the student gets yelled at!! But finally, when the coach throws everything he has at his student, and not only does he withstand the beating, but he knocks the coach down, there is nobody in the world happier than the coach himself!

This is exactly how I feel. If you fail right away and don't even try to fight back, I see that there is not much talent to work with, and so I take it easy on you. But if you get back up swinging, I realize that I may have a real winner here, so I start to intensify the beating. With every level that you go up, I increase the intensity of the fight. If you finally deal me a blow that knocks me out, I will get up and embrace you and rejoice in your success.

Sometimes my job is very disappointing. I see a person with a lot of potential, and I start right in on him. He fights back for a while, but he quits and remains on whatever level he is on when the fight gets too tough. (And he usually ends up going down!) I feel like yelling at him, "Get up, you fool! Do you have any idea how much more you could be accomplishing?" But I am not allowed to do so.

I leave him alone and go try to find another promising candidate. If I have chosen you to be the target of my fierce battles, it was not for no reason! You have a tremendous ability! You were born into an exceptional family; you have Rabbeim who care about you and parents who would help you grow in Torah and Mitzvot. You are a very respectful and kind person. I am writing to you now because I have an earnest request to ask of you. Please don't stop fighting! Don't give up! I have been beating too many people lately, and I am losing patience. Believe in yourself because I would not be involved with you as much as I am if I didn't think you could beat me. Know what your strength is! A great rabbi once said, "Woe is to him who doesn't know his weaknesses. But, 'Oy Vavoy' to him who doesn't know his strengths—for he will not have anything with which to fight."

Always remember one thing: you have a secret weapon at your disposal. I shouldn't be telling you, but I will anyway. Hashem Himself is watching our "training" sessions very closely. I'm pleased to inform you that he's rooting for you! If things should ever get too tough to bear, call out to Him with a prayer, and He will immediately come to your aid. I wish you the best of luck, and I hope that after 120 years, when your time is up in that world of falsehood, you will come up here to the world of truth, where I will be waiting for you with open arms to congratulate you on your victory, and personally escort you to your place next to the Kisei HaKavod. Sincerely and with great admiration, I remain your Yetzer Hara.

9) Righteous Warriors (By Rebbe Lazer Brody Shalita)

Righteous Warriors (from a lecture from the Esteemed Rav Lazer Brody Shalita)

There are great masters and leaders of our past who showed skill as scholars, prophets, and kings, and as physical warriors. This indicates that when we build our minds and spirits, we are also preparing Our bodies (in the event of war, strife, or protection of the innocent, and more).

Bible Period

Abraham: The first Jew defeated the superpower of his day (Nimrod and four other kings) with a small band of 318 soldiers.

Simon and Levi: Sons of Jacob. At age thirteen, they wiped out a Canaanite city whose prince forcibly abducted their sister, Dina.

Joshua: Moses's protégé. Defeated the armies of the Amalek and Canaanite nations and also executed a dangerous espionage mission in Jericho.

King David: As a shepherd, before his Bar Mitzvah, he killed a lion and a bear that tried to seize his sheep. At age twelve, he killed the evil Goliath. King David was not only a holy man and the Almighty's anointed author of the Book of Psalms; he was a pro in archery, fencing, and hand-to-hand combat.

Second Temple Period

Yehuda ben Mattityahu (the Maccabee): A brilliant Torah scholar and fierce warrior, he drove the entire Greek army out of Israel.

Talmudic Period

Rabbi Simon Ben Lakish (RESH LAKISH): Forced by the Romans to become a gladiator, he indeed killed lions in the arena. Later, when kidnapped by ten massive cannibals of the Ludim tribe, he disposed of them with his bare hands.

The Holocaust

The Radziner Rebbe: The hero of the Warsaw Ghetto, who fearlessly fought the evil Nazis.

The secret to winning like the men of old

1. Fear GOD when you have a real fear of GOD; nothing in the world can shake you.

2. Love GOD. When you love GOD, you have faith (Emunah) that he will protect you.

3. If you want to succeed either in ancient fighting techniques or today's martial arts, learn Talmud. The Talmud will teach you how to concentrate. Concentration and focus are essential in physical

training. The direction of energy and focus on movement can be sharpened with Torah learning. You, too, can be a righteous warrior!

10) Thankfulness

Often, the Yetzer Hara (animal or evil inclination) will attempt to bring us down by attacking our minds with worry, doubt, anxiety, stress, and more. So, to fight and win against these experiences that come to attack us daily, it is important to stay thankful. Here is an exercise that can help.

Grab a pen and use the following few pages to write down all the things GOD has blessed you with. The more specific you are, the better. There is no time like the present, so start your list! Example:

- Being able to wake up each morning.
- Being able to get out of bed.
- Having my eyes work.
- Having my arms and legs work.
- Being able to hear from both ears and not just one or neither.
- Having a family member.
- Having a friend.
- Having a hobby.
- Having a place to pray.
- Food on the table, etc.
- Longevity.

Below are some great tips to help us live a longer and more meaningful life. Dr. Shmuel Shields, Ph.D., asked a woman who had reached her 100th birthday her secret for longevity.

Here are her points:

- Love yourself
- Think positively
- Hold yourself in high esteem
- Exercise every day (even if it's a 15-20-minute walk)
- Say "No" to negative thoughts
- Love life
- Make every day count
- Have love in your heart for everyone
- If you want a friend, you have to be a friend
- Enjoy your own company.
- It is important to you.
- Keep smiling

11) Torah-Based Longevity Tips

Here are some guidelines for longevity based on Torah and Talmudic sources (by Dr. Shmuel Shields)

- "Honor your father and mother" (Shemot 20:12).
- "Send away a mother bird before removing her eggs." (Devarim 22:7)
- "Arrive early and stay late in shul." (Berachos 8a)
- "Refrain from displaying impatience or anger at home."

(Taanis 20b; Megillah 28a)

- "Do not neglect to say Kiddush on Shabbat." (Megillah 27b)
- "Do not use shul/synagogue as a shortcut [just to get someplace else]." (Megillah 28a)
- "Forgive anyone who aggravates you" (Megillah 28a). "Be wise, yet liberal with your money in giving to others."
- (Megillah 28a) Breakfast of Spiritual and Physical Champions!

What is "Machalah"? It means sickness or sickness in the whole human body. Machalah is also numerically 83, and Gemara, Bava Metziah, 107b says that seventy-three illnesses are dependent upon the gall. All of them may be rendered harmless by eating one's morning bread with salt and drinking a jug full of water. Our rabbis taught thirteen.

Things were said of the morning bread:

It is an antidote against heat (in the summer) and cold (in the winter), winds and demons; it instills wisdom into the simple (by being satiated he is tranquil and thus can study better), causes one to triumph in a lawsuit (his tranquility causes him to state his case better), enables one to study and teach the Torah, to have his words heeded (tranquility renders eloquence), and retain scholarship; he (who partakes of it) does not perspire, lives with his wife, and does not lust after other women; and it kills the worms in one's intestines. Some say it also expels jealousy and induces love (for fellow humans, i.e., a hungry man upset early). Rabbah asked Rava bar Mari, "From where comes the proverbial expression, 'Sixty runners speed along, but cannot overtake him who breaks bread in the morning,' and also the Rabbinical dictum,

"Arise early and eat in the summer, on account of the heat, and in the winter, on account of the cold." He replied, "Because it is written, 'They shall not hunger or thirst; neither shall the cold nor sun smite them.'"

"(Isaiah 49:10) Thus, "the cold or sun shall not smite them, "because they shall neither hunger nor thirst." He said to him, "You deduce it from that verse, but I, from this: "You will serve the Lord your GOD, and He will (thereby) bless your food and your water (and I shall remove illness from your midst). "You will serve the Lord your GOD." This refers to the reading of the Shema and prayer, "and He will (thereby) bless your food and your water," to bread and salt, and to a jug of water. Afterward, I shall remove illness from your Midst.

WOW! I was shocked when I heard this as well. So many benefits to breaking bread in the morning! Amazing stuff. So, to sum it up, of course, with washing hands and saying Hamotz, I have breakfast. We asked our rabbi, and he advised us to have water before and say the Shehakol blessing on the water, then rinse. Also, he said if someone is having trouble and can't have bread, he can have a baked grain product, but the best way is to have the bread; you can also go with whole wheat if you like to have this on a more frequent basis. So, of course, you can get as creative as you wish; maybe make an avocado toast sandwich with lemon, olive oil, and salt, or perhaps a toast with banana and blueberry with almond butter or tahini. If you like sweets, throw a little date syrup or honey on top, and don't forget the blessing of Birkat Hamazon! Enjoy. Summary: One should make a point to eat every morning either bread or other baked grain products, in a quantity of at least 2 oz. "Be bold as a leopard." The piece below is derived from Halachayomit.com regarding the Mishna.

The Mishnah in Pirkei Avot (Chapter 5) states, "Yehuda ben Tema says, 'Be bold like a leopard, light as an eagle, swift as a deer, and mighty as a lion to perform the will of your Father in Heaven." Let us now explain this: Mishnah. The Tanna writes that one must be as "bold as a leopard," meaning that there are times when one will abstain from performing a mitzvah because others ridicule him. The Mishnah, therefore, commands not to refrain from performing the Mitzvot under any circumstances; rather, one must be bold in the face.

Of those who ridicule him and perform the mitzvot. This is especially relevant regarding things that society is not accustomed to. For instance, if a woman has friends who do not cover their hair, it will be very difficult for her to cover her hair, for she will be afraid to lose her friends. Similarly, if one wishes not to lose out on his daily Torah class and therefore decides not to answer his phone during classes, he will be afraid that his friends will ridicule him and that he "has become a righteous fellow." Another example is when one wishes not to speak during prayer services and his friend, sitting next to him, asks him a question. Again, one will undoubtedly be ashamed not to answer. In all these and similar situations, one must be bold and unswerving to keep the commandments of Hashem as one wishes. Thus, Hashem will help make an individual more admired by his peers for his commitment to Torah and mitzvot.

Nevertheless, one must take great care not to fight with others, for ultimately, boldness and audacity are bad traits, so much so that some say they should not even be used for the service of Hashem. Therefore, one should secure for himself friends and acquaintances of high spiritual caliber who are Torah and mitzvot observant themselves to ease one's commitment to Judaism.

The Mishnah states specifically, "light like an eagle," instead of any other bird, because the eagle has extraordinary sight even at great distances. Although it flies at great altitudes, it can discern any carcass on the ground. Our Sages, therefore, warn us to be cautious regarding what our eyes see, for sight is the first stage of sinning since the eyes see, the heart desires, and the other limbs achieve the Sin. Instead, one must be as "light as an eagle" and quickly ignore what one has seen and what one's heart desires.

When the Mishnah states that one must be "swift like a deer," this refers to the fact that one's legs should always run to good things, as King David states (Tehillim 119), "Guide me in the path of your commandments." One should not become lethargic while on their way to perform a Mitzvah. When the Mishnah states that one must be as "mighty as a lion," this teaches us that one must be as mighty as a lion regarding the performance of the Mitzvot. Therefore, one must overcome his evil inclination and abstain from performing prohibitions, for both performing Mitzvot and abstaining from sinning require tremendous might. Based on this, Maran begins the first chapter of his Shulchan. Aruch as follows:

"One must infuse himself with might like a lion to awaken in the morning to the service of his Creator, and one should awaken even before dawn." The Poskim explain that if one cannot wake up so early in the morning, especially nowadays, when we have electricity and therefore do not go to sleep as early, or if one is worried that waking up so early will disturb his Torah study and service of Hashem, according to the letter of the law, one may wake up later. One must nevertheless take care not to miss the latest times for reciting Keriat Shema and prayer, for one is obligated to abide by these times. One must always think to himself how careful one would be to arise early if he were commanded to serve a king of flesh and blood; how much more so must one take care regarding the service of the King of all Kings, Hashem, blessed is He?

SECTION V

CONCLUSION

I commend you for taking steps to get to this point. But, just like any worthy challenge or mission, you have to make a sacrifice, maybe take some hits, and commit yourself to a goal. As you know, success is difficult, but it is doable and lasting with GOD's blessings. This program aims to help you find spiritual truth and give you tools and tips for wellness goals.

We humbly lay out information and tools to help you find answers for yourself because you are worth it! We are not adrift in a universe caused by chance but fellow citizens of this island universe and fellow voyagers on the beautiful blue sphere called Earth, floating through space and time. The absolute miracle of life is the indisputable fact that on our planet, home to seven billion humans, there are, possibly with only a slight variation, billions of hearts beating because Hashem has allowed it.

No more complaining, worrying, or living in the past. Start being present and thankful each morning; you are blessed to wake up and have a shot at the world. Now is your time. There are no more excuses. You currently have more than enough information and tools. Refer to your thankfulness list any time you feel down. Be mindful of your environment and pay attention to your feelings and your mind.

Find a friend and a rabbi and go to nature and talk to GOD when you need someone to talk to. Be happy, live, and love yourself!! You're amazing and made in the image of GOD.

Please try to learn more than provided in this book, like reading the Written and Oral Torah and Joining an Orthodox Torah class in your local community or online. If you are not ready, you can contact Soulfit.com for advice and/or tips depending on your situation. Gaining additional knowledge is never a waste. You will find new ideas and creative ways to begin a new life characterized by robust physical and spiritual well-being.

In Aryeh Kaplan's (with Rabbi Sutton) book Inner Space, the Talmudic statement says that GOD will take the Yetzer Hara (Evil Urge) and ritually slaughter it in the ultimate future. The Holy Baal Shem Tov asks why Yetzer Hara, the entire realm of evil, deserves to be killed. Despite appearances to the contrary, is it God's faithful servant? The Baal Shem Tov points out that it does not say that GOD will kill the Yetzer Hara but slaughter it. When certain animals are slaughtered ritually, they are made kosher. The slaughtering of the Yetzer Hara in the world to come means that GOD will make him into a good angel.

The world to come is a dimension of ultimate reward and closeness to GOD when the period of testing for humankind will come to a close, and the very concept of evil will no longer be necessary.

At that time, GOD will rectify evil itself and return it to its root. In the meantime, the realm of evil is needed to tempt us and give us free will and free choice to maximize the struggle and the challenge of serving GOD in this world. For this to occur, however, an interface is needed for evil to draw its nourishment from the Divine. Some mechanisms whereby the Divine can interact with evil and give the power to function. Second, one needs protection so that evil does not have the power to blemish the realm of the Holy Way.

This should give you the clarity to prepare for the end of days and stay motivated to learn the Torah, do more mitzvot, and stay holy. To help even further, we must remember the lesson in Purim that we need to reach a level where we realize there is no difference between Mordechai Hatzaik and Haman Harasha. The good guys and bad guys (Hashem is running the show) are all the same! Super hard level to reach, but a vision and mindset to attain.

Remember, the end will not be easy. The test will be the hardest, just like Pharaoh increased the labor and workload with taskmasters; the end of the exile will be more complex and more challenging, but that just means we are closer and closer to redemption, so hold on tight, we are almost there! You don't need any more stats and fancy graphs. Our "Tzadikim have paved the way for us," and in their merit the world continues to exist. See proof in Gemara in Chullin 92a and Gemara in Sukkah 45b. We must attach and be close to real Tzadikim of this generation and of past generations (by learning their books, etc.). We must strive to have Emunah in Hashem and his Tzadikim in a simple manner. We only included information from non-Jewish sources earlier in the book for those not yet on level, but once you have it, you will see you won't need it. The Tzadikim have helped us. The simple faith is perhaps the most sophisticated and highest level of wisdom.

Thank you so much for taking this journey with our handbook. We look forward to celebrating at the third and final temple in Jerusalem! Please document and date your progress so you can always look back and feel great about where you started. It is all up to you!

We will end with a quote from the Prophet Isaiah to illustrate the new world of peace and happiness that will soon come to our planet with the Mashiach (Messiah):

"In the days to come, the mountain of GOD's house shall stand firm above the mountains and tower above the hills. And all the nations shall stream to it. And the many peoples shall go and say, 'Come, let us go up to the Mount of GOD, to the House of the GOD of Jacob— that He may instruct us in His ways, that we may walk in His paths. And they shall beat their swords into plowshares and their spears into pruning hooks; nation shall not lift sword against nation.

Neither shall they learn war anymore; at that time, the wolf shall dwell with the lamb, the leopard will lie down with the kid, and the calf and beast of prey shall feed together with a little child to herd them.

APPENDIX

APPENDIX A:

THE RAMBAN'S LETTER

The great champion Rabbi Moses ben Nachman Gerondi, known by the abbreviation Ramban, wrote to his elder son, Nachman, instructing him to read it weekly.

Hear, my son, the instruction of your father, and do not forsake the teaching of your mother (Mishlei 1:8). Get into the habit of always speaking calmly to everyone. This will prevent you from anger, a serious character flaw that causes people to sin. As our rabbis said (Nedarim 22a):

Whoever flares up in anger is subject to the discipline of Gehinnom, as it is said in Kohelet 12:10, "Cast out anger from your heart, and [by doing this] remove evil from your flesh." "Evil" here means Gehinnom, as we read (Mishlei 16:4): "... and the wicked are destined for the day of evil." Once you have distanced yourself from anger, the quality of humility will enter your heart.

This radiant quality is the finest of all admirable traits (see Avodah Zarah 20b) because (Mishlei 22:4), "Following humility comes the fear of Hashem."

Through humility, you will also come to fear Hashem. It will cause you to always think about (see Avos 3:1) where you came from and where you are going, and that while alive, you are only like a maggot and a worm, and the same after death.

It will also remind you before whom you will be judged, the King of Glory, as it is stated (I Melachim 8:27; Mishlei 15:11), "Even the heaven and the heavens of heaven cannot contain You"—"How much less the hearts of people!" It is also written (Yirmeyahu 23:24), "Do I not fill heaven and earth? says Hashem."

When you think about all these things, you will come to fear Hashem, who created you, and you will protect yourself from sinning and, therefore, be happy with whatever happens to you. Also, when you act humbly and modestly before everyone and are afraid of Hashem and sin, the radiance of His glory and the spirit of the Shechina will rest upon you, and you will live the life of the World to Come!

And now, my son, understand and observe that whoever feels that he is greater than others is rebelling against the Kingship of Hashem because he is adorning himself with His garments, as it is written (Tehillim 93:1), "Hashem reigns; He wears clothes of pride." Why should one feel proud? Is it because of wealth?

Hashem makes one poor or rich (I Shmuel 2:7). Is it because of honor? It belongs to Hashem, as we read (Divrei Hayamim 29:12), "Wealth and honor come from You." So how could one adorn himself with Hashem's honor? And one who is proud of his wisdom surely knows that Hashem "takes away the speech of assured men and reasoning from the sages" (Iyov 12:20)!? We see that everyone is the same before Hashem since, with His anger, He lowers the pride, and when He wishes, He raises the low. So, lower yourself, and Hashem will lift you!

I will now explain to you how to always behave humbly. Speak gently at all times, with your head bowed, your eyes looking down to the ground, and your heart focusing on Hashem. Do not look at the face of the person to whom you are speaking. Consider everyone as greater than yourself. If he is wise or rich, you should give him respect. If he is poor and you are wealthier or wiser than he, consider yourself to be guiltier than he, and that he is worthier than you, since when he sins, it is through error, while yours is deliberate, and you should know better! In all your actions, words, and thoughts, always regard yourself as standing before Hashem, with His Shechinah above you, for His glory fills the whole world. Speak with fear and awe as a slave standing before his master. Act with restraint in front of everyone.

When someone calls you, do not answer loudly, but gently and softly, as one who stands before his master. The Torah should always be learned diligently, so you will be able to fulfill its commands. When you arise from your learning, reflect carefully on what you have studied to see what you can put into practice. Examine your actions every morning and evening, and in this way, every one of your days will be spent in teshuvah (repentance).

Concentrate on your prayers by removing all worldly concerns from your heart. Prepare your heart before Hashem, purify your thoughts, and think about what you are going to say. If you follow this in all your daily actions, you will not come to sin.

This way, everything you do will be proper, and your prayer will be pure, clear, clean, devout, and acceptable to Hashem, as it is written (Tehillim 10:17), "When their heart is directed to You, listen to them."

Read this letter at least once a week and neglect none of it. Fulfill it, and in so doing, walk with it forever in the ways of Hashem; may he be blessed so that you will succeed in all your ways. Thus, you will succeed and merit the world to come, which lies hidden away for the righteous. Every day that you shall read this letter, heaven shall answer your heart's desires. Amen, Sela!

APPENDIX B:

KASHRUTH, YOUR SPIRITUAL ANTENNA

I am sure you have listened to an AM radio station, and the signal is very weak, and you can hardly hear the station. Well, for righteous Yehudim, this is the best analogy I can come up with. Eating kosher will increase the signal to your spiritual antenna. For our righteous Noahide friends, there is no obligation to eat kosher (Gentiles need to keep the 7 Noahide laws), but you can read more about it below. So, for you, righteous Yehudim, continue reading. Keeping kosher and putting on tefillin can be a perfect step in your journey.

So, what exactly do we mean by eating kosher? What sets kosher foods apart from all the other types of food and food preparation? Does eating kosher help all persons in the quest for glowing health? Although eating kosher was originally intended only for those Torah-observant Jews who keep all the commandments, its dietary system has been validated by science in recent years, and if so, how could eating kosher benefit you even if you are not Jewish?

Kosher, also known as kashrut, is a term that refers to the types of food that may be eaten according to the Torah and also to the acceptable ways in which they may be prepared. Although, unfortunately, many think that the meaning of kosher is limited only to food types, in contrast, food is essential in understanding what is

And what is not truly kosher. It is not the only deciding factor. For example, in meat(s), the animal must be slaughtered as quickly and humanely as possible to reduce the animal's suffering. This shows the sensitivity and care of the beautiful animal kingdom. "Kosher" can also refer to acceptable drinks such as wine and milk. All the steps in the act of eating are instinctual, as they are wonderfully simple. However, for those who follow the Torah, the act of eating is no longer solely driven by instinct, but mind, spirit, and soul start to play a decisive role in how we take in nourishment as well.

To understand better what the Torah says about eating as a mindful and sacred activity, consider what the Jewish tradition says about the basics of "keeping kosher." First, all animals or birds eating meat must be free of seventy different types of disease, injury, or other conditions unsafe for human consumption. In short, they must not be what is known in Yiddish as treif. Any animal considered kosher must chew its cud, which is best defined as "food regurgitated from the first stomach to the mouth of a ruminant and chewed again." Animals that chew their cud are also known as ruminants, the most prominent being cattle, sheep, goats, deer, etc.

Therefore, this class of ruminants is quite exclusive. Animals such as dogs, bears, pigs, etc., do not fall into the kashrut category, but common fowls such as chickens, ducks, and geese do. Not all birds of prey are kosher; hence, falcons, hawks, and owls are "unclean."

Not just mammals, but the members of the bird family that are permitted to be eaten must also be slaughtered as humanely, painlessly, and quickly as possible. Only a surgically sharp knife may be used to cut the animal's trachea, esophagus, carotid artery, and jugular vein. This fast action, which requires a precisely sharp knife, automatically sends the blood pressure in the brain to zero, so the bird loses consciousness instantly and dies in minutes. In the interests of humaneness, a "kid [baby calf or goat] must not be boiled in its mother's milk." This was a common practice in the days of the Canaanites when Moses was trying hard to civilize the Israelites before Hashem would permit them entrance into the Promised Land, "a land overflowing with milk and honey."

Before GOD would allow them a surfeit of food and prosperity, He demanded that Moses cause them to cease all such cruel acts against animals reserved for food. Perhaps in 1871 the cruelest act of all was eating both the mother and its kid together in a devil's brew, such as basting the calf in its own mother's milk. To never commit such a heinous act against a calf, the Torah leads the observant Jew light-years away from such a possibility, only by prohibiting the mixing together (on any level).

The Torah calls the Jews a "holy people" and prescribes a holy diet (see Deut. 14:24). You are what you eat. Kosher is GOD's diet for spirituality. Jewish mysticism teaches that nonkosher food blocks the spiritual potential of the soul.

Kosher animals properly slaughtered and prepared have more "sparks of holiness" (according to the Kabbalah) incorporated into

Our being. If a person can be disciplined in what and when he eats, he can be disciplined in other areas of life. For example, Kashrut requires that one wait after eating meat before eating milk products, and we may not eat certain animals or combinations of foods. (Even when you are hungry!) All of this instills self-discipline.

If you disagree with these understandings and benefits, that is okay, too. Because the real reason we eat kosher is that GOD commanded us to do so in the Torah, and the Jewish people are bound to GOD by a covenant to keep the commandments of the Torah. To learn more about kashrut, read "The Kosher Kitchen" by Rabbi Ze'ev Greenwald, a user-friendly, practical, and illustrated guide that eliminates the mystery and confusion of keeping kosher.

Of course, the Almighty does not want us to become neurotic. If one wants to upgrade his observance of the Torah, it should be done in intelligent, calculated steps. Just as a parent loves the first steps of a toddler, the Almighty treasures our steps toward fulfilling His Torah. Do what you can, with thoughts of doing even more.

APPENDIX C:

HARAV'S PROCESS OVERVIEW:

Below is great wisdom from my own personal Rabbi Netaneli Shalita
Core Concept: Harav recommends taking on a mitzvah that is challenging for an individual, suggesting that by choosing specific hardships, one can avoid or mitigate other life difficulties.

Mechanism:

The hardship from mitzvot fills one's life, leaving no room for additional, naturally occurring hardships. Over time, this mitzvah becomes sweet and enjoyable.

Implementation:

When facing difficulty in the chosen mitzvah, one should pray for relief in other areas of life. Harav blesses individuals, suggesting that through this mitzvah, salvation will come, without specifying why difficulties arise.

Specific Mitzvot and Practices:

General Recommendations:

Shabbat and Kosher: Essential for those not yet observing these commandments.

For Married Women:

Head Covering:

Advised to cover hair fully with a scarf, not a wig, for reasons discussed here: https://malachei26.com/book1/#flipbook_df_811/3/ This practice is believed to bring peace, health, and prosperity to the home.

Blessings and Eating:

Before and After Eating:

Say blessings like Mezonot, Haetz, Haadama, and Shehakol with full concentration. Birkat Hamazon should be said with clear enunciation, not rushed.

Hand Washing Before Bread: Wash hands three times alternately, followed by a blessing if consuming 50 grams or more of bread.

Morning Rituals:

Netilat Yadayim at Bedside:

Harav emphasizes its importance for removing negative energy ("Ruach Ra'a"). Instructions:

Prepare a cup of water by the bed before sleep.

Wash your hands before your feet touch the ground in the morning.

-   Use water prepared outside the bathroom, **not left uncovered overnight.**

After the initial washing, no blessing is said until after using the restroom; then wash again and say blessings ("Al Netilat Yadayim" and "Asher Yatzar") using a sink outside the bathroom.

Video explaining how to pour the water:

Rabbi Eliyahu Netaneli

Demonstrating Morning Netilat Yadayim

🎥 Video https://MyTAT.me/v42553

For Men:

Torah Study:

Recommended to study "Hok L'Yisrael," which includes Torah and Targum commentary on the weekly Parasha. | Chok L'Yisrael

General Spiritual Advice:

Focus During Blessings: Stand still and concentrate fully when speaking to God.

Spiritual Purity: Ensures protection against negative energy or the evil eye (Ayin Hara).

Prayer for Healing:

Something powerful you can do is read **Tehillim 119** in a special order. Chapter 119 is arranged using every letter in the Hebrew alphabet. Each paragraph starts with a corresponding Hebrew letter in **רפוא שלמה**order. Find the letters of his name followed by the word and read those chapters in order of those letters. Do not speak once Just the letters below. It is very .(בן) started, and do not do the letters powerful.

יהודה רפואה סיון חיה רפוא שלמה

Inspirational first-hand miracle stories:

https://vimeo.com/showcase/10508324

Many physical ailments or difficulties in our lives stem from a spiritual void or deficiency. Harav systematically reviews essential spiritual practices to identify where a physical or life blockage might originate, whether it's related to health, finances, or marriage. He believes that by committing to a challenging mitzvah, one invokes Hashem's mercy, potentially alleviating hardships in other areas of life. By choosing to strictly adhere to a Torah law, we can, in essence, select our challenges, hoping this will mitigate those difficulties beyond our control.

APPENDIX D:

COLLECTIVE AND PERSONAL GUELLA

The journey to Geulah isn't just about waiting; it's about actively bringing it closer, and one of the most powerful ways to do that is through how we see and treat each other. Ahavat Yisrael (loving our fellow Jew) is not just a nice idea—it's foundational to Torah and maybe the ultimate key to hastening both our collective and your personal Geulah.

1. Rabbi Moshe Cordovero (Ramak)—Seeing the Holiness in Every Jew

Rabbi Moshe Cordovero, one of the great Kabbalists of Tzfat (16th century), taught that if you see a Jew sin or appear distant from holiness, never judge them negatively. Instead, immediately remind yourself: their ancestors were holy, and their neshama is rooted in the same kedusha as yours. This means they, too, have an inherent holiness, even if it's currently hidden. Love them, see them favorably, and daven for them.

Source: Tomer Devorah, Chapter 2—A person must cultivate the attribute of Hashem, who always sees the potential for good and never permanently rejects His children.

2. Rabbi Chaim Vital—Love Your Fellow as Yourself Before Praying

Rabbi Chaim Vital in Pri Etz Chaim discusses the teachings of his Rebbi, the Arizal, that before beginning to daven each morning, a person should explicitly accept upon themselves the mitzvah of "Ve'ahavta L'reiacha Kamocha"—loving every Jew as oneself. This is not a mere formality; it changes the way our tefillot are received. The Magen Avraham, a major halachic authority, even noted how this custom became widespread due to its Kabbalistic significance.

Sources: Pri Etz Chaim, Sha'ar HaTefillah, Ch. 2; Magen Avraham Orach Chaim 46:8 – The Arizal emphasized that unity among Jews is a necessary prerequisite for proper prayer.

3. The Baal Shem Tov—The World is a Mirror

The Baal Shem Tov (founder of Chassidus, 17th century) revealed a deep secret: if you see another Jew sin, don't rush to judge. Instead, understand that Hashem is showing you your own flaws reflected at you. The world is a mirror—when we notice faults in others, it's often a sign that we need to do teshuvah ourselves.

Just like a parent sees their own traits mirrored in their children (especially before a bar/bat mitzvah), our reality reflects what's inside us. Change yourself, and you'll see others start to change as well.

Sources: Keter Shem Tov, 69; Tzava'at HaRivash—"One "who judges others favorably creates merit not just for them, but for themselves."

4. Rabbi Levi Yitzchak of Berdichev—The Defender of Am Yisrael

Rabbi Levi Yitzchak of Berdichev (17th/18th century) was known as the greatest advocate of the Jewish people. He never stopped defending them, even when they strayed. If you see a Jew sinning, don't write them off; pray for them, defend them, and assume they may not fully understand what they are doing.

Many times, people simply forget, don't know, or are temporarily overwhelmed by the yetzer hara. Keep this perspective in mind and in your heart, because just as we want Hashem to judge us favorably, we must judge others the same way. Sources: Kedushat Levi, Parshat Vayeishev – Hashem desires an advocate for His people, not a prosecutor.

The Balance: Love the Uninformed, Oppose the Corrupt
While we are obligated to love and uplift every Jew, there's a critical distinction to be made:

- If someone is simply unlearned or has never had the chance to grow in Torah, our responsibility is to embrace them, teach them, and guide them with love.

- But if someone knows the Torah and deliberately fights against it, misleading others, we have a duty to oppose their influence. This includes so-called "leaders" or, unfortunately, maybe some people who use the title "rabbi" who promote falsehood.

We must stand for truth and ensure that we and others are not led astray.

This is not a contradiction; it's part of the same principle. We uplift those who lack knowledge, and we protect the integrity of the Torah from those who distort it.

Sources: Rambam, Hilchot De'ot 6:7—One must distance oneself from a deliberate sinner who influences others negatively.

In summary, Geulah begins when we see each other the way Hashem sees us—with love, with hope, and with the belief that every Jew can return. It's not always easy, but it's our mission. By applying these lessons, we don't just bring light to others—we bring light to ourselves and to the world. And with Hashem's help, that light will soon become the full radiance of Mashiach; may we be zocheh to see it speedily in our days.

5) Rabbi Nachman of Uman- Tzadik Yesod Olam

Rebbe Nachman is a unique figure in the history of Chassidut, the Jewish revival movement founded by his great-grandfather, the Baal Shem Tov (Master of the Good Name). In his lifetime, the Rebbe was well-known as a Chassidic master, attracting hundreds of followers. Today, over 200 years after his passing, his following numbers in the tens of thousands, making him a vibrant source of encouragement and guidance in today's world. Rebbe in 1772, twelve years after the Baal Shem Tov's passing, in the western Ukrainian town of Medzeboz. The Rebbe had two brothers and a sister. During his childhood, many Chassidic masters would come to visit the grave of the Baal Shem Tov in Medzeboz and they would stay in the Rebbe's parents house. Rebbe Nachman was deeply inspired by these great leaders to become an outstanding Tzaddik and Torah sage himself. He acquired his first disciple on his wedding day in 1785. After his marriage he moved to the eastern Ukrainian town of Ossatin. In the early 1790s he moved to nearby Medvedevka, where he began to attract a devoted following. In 1798-1799, at the height of the Napoleonic wars in the Middle East, he made his pilgrimage to the Holy Land.

Know! you must judge all people favorably. Even in the case of a complete sinner, you must search until you find some good in him!

Rebbe Nachman teaches: Know! you must judge all people favorably. Even in the case of a complete sinner, you must search until you find some good in him, some small aspect in which he is not a sinner. Buy doing this, you actually elevate him to the side of merit. You can then bring him to return to God. This can be understood from the verse, "In but a *little bit* the sinner is not; search carefully his place and he is not there" (Psalms 37:10). If you find but a little bit of good, then the sinner is not – he is no longer guilty; search his place and he is not there – but is now to be found on the side of merit (*Likutey Moharan* I, 282).

So begins Rebbe Nachman's lesson *AZAMRA!* Conceivably the most important lesson in all of *Likutey Moharan*, it is the only one which carries the Rebbe's exhortation: "Go with this lesson, constantly!" Keep it in mind and practice it, always! (The publication *AZAMRA!* contains the entire lesson and Reb Noson's commentary in translation, explaining these concepts at length.) Why is the message of this lesson so special?

"...If you find but a little bit of good, then the sinner is not – he is no longer guilty; search his place and he is not there – but is now to be found on the side of merit!" (Likutey Moharan I, 282).

The faculty of judgement is one of man's most powerful tools. If we really knew just how potent, we would certainly be more careful about how we used it. Elsewhere, the Rebbe teaches that judging others can destroy the world. If a person finds fault with another, this judgment can condemn him (*Likutey Moharan* I, 3). Think about it! your evaluation, your opinion and judgement of others has the power to either elevate or degrade.

The problem is that criticism comes easy. Too easy. We can always find fault in what others do or fail to do. It's not difficult to ascribe ulterior motives even for the worthiest of deeds. This is especially true when we hear slander. Then everyone is quick to jump on the bandwagon condemning the offender for his wrongdoing. We have to realize that every word spoken about another person is, in some way, a form of judgment. If, in our judgment, we find the good points and focus on the positive, we can bring the world – the entire world – to the side of merit and worthiness. However, the reverse is also true. In judging others, if we find fault and focus on the negative, we can bring the world – the entire world – to the side of demerit and unworthiness. This is why we must always try to look for the good in others, even in the worst person we know. Such emphasis on his positive traits affects him, because, as Rebbe Nachman said, our favorable judgment "actually elevates him to the side of merit."

Sources: Judge everybody favorably! (*Avot* 1:6). This promotes peace (Rashi).

One who judges others favorably, is himself judged favorably (*Shabbat* 127b).

God's way is to focus on the good. Even if there are things which are not so good, He only looks for the good. How much more do we have to avoid focusing on the faults of our friends. We are obligated to seek only the good – always! (*Likutey Moharan* II, 17).

APPENDIX E:

"THE FAB 5" By Rebbi Meir Elkabas

Get out of the darkness/sadness mode in 4 minutes or less!
There is no *yeush* (no giving up on yourself).

1. Jokes / Silliness

Tell some kosher jokes, even corny ones, just to snap out of the sadness mode quickly. A little humor helps shift your mind one step closer to a better place than before. Acting a little silly (of course, not crazy, just a little) can help shift your mind and body to a more positive state.

2. Dancing and Music

Put on some kosher music, acappella, Breslev, Chassidic, etc. It helps move us toward the light faster. Clap your hands, move your feet; real lasting joy is found in dancing. Even if you don't feel like it, try to push yourself. You'll feel good later. Clap, dance, or do any moves you like. Yes, you've got it!

3. Azamra!

Look at the good points in yourself. Yes, you're amazing. You are a son/daughter of the King, the Creator of everything. Even in what seems like "bad" or tough times, try to find **one** good point in yourself. This will, b'ezrat Hashem, help you fix things much faster.

4. Hodaya! (Giving Thanks—Quick Lesson)

When we say *Modeh Ani* while still in bed, we see that the Torah allows us to speak to Hashem before *netilat yadayim* (in an impure moment) because of the importance of gratitude. Within thankfulness, the blessings of the day are hidden. Still, we strive to wash our hands as quickly as possible, preferably near the bed.

5. Envision the Future

The Third Temple, the resurrection of the dead, and the punishment of the wicked. Good will prevail! Can't wait. Hope to see you there with all our ancestors. Yes, we're all one family.

Point number 5 is brought down as something to do if one has trouble falling asleep.

You don't need to be extreme—stay normal, stay healthy, stay happy.

These five tips can help you quickly get out of "sadness" or "dark" moments in your car, at work, or in your room.

Rabbi Nachman of Breslev explains the deep importance of being happy.

It has a powerful spiritual element: when you work on these points, you can return sparks and lost objects that belong to you (and others) from the "Exchange Chambers." To learn more about this, request to Rebbi Meir to be added to his group. Rabbi Meir is available on whats app 1(732) 800-1863

ABOUT THE AUTHOR

Growing up in Los Angeles, Baruch Hashem was filled with its own B'H' (challenges). I grew up in both the Jewish Orthodox and public school systems. I saw both worlds, but of course, as a child and in a home that was filled with faith but a bit far from having all Torah Mitzvot in place , playing sports. As a result, I developed a passion for sports and tried my hand at several sporting activities.

We started in the Jewish school system but then moved to the public school system with my parents' divorce, and it unsettled me a bit. Nonetheless, I always kept what I learned from my parents and my Jewish faith. I started to take a strong enjoyment in the kids playing basketball, and that helped me with my emotions. When things seemed "dark," I spent all my spare time playing outdoors and more into the game of basketball. Which began to grow with me. I knew if I ever wanted to make the school's team, I had to work hard and try to perfect my craft.

I began familiarizing myself with the theoretical aspects of the game and learning the sport's history from the farms of Indiana to the streets of New York. I enjoyed playing, but soon, in high school, I Appreciated the philosophy and psychology of what it takes to coach yourself and others to be the best you can be.

Eventually, I made it to the school varsity team and soon became the team's captain. After high school, I was humbled to make it into a

Division 1 university. It was like a dream to travel to various top colleges in America and play against some of the best players in the world while I was just 18 years old. I toured different cities, stadiums, and tournaments, participating in many competitions and tournaments with sometimes over 10,000 spectators in attendance.

Combining sports and religion was interesting for me as I joined the team's Bible study class. Interestingly, I initially rebuffed an invitation to the Bible study class, citing my Jewish faith as a reason. I was reminded by a teammate who told me, "Yes, JC was Jewish, [so] you can come," but I remained steadfast in my resolve not to take part. However, as the years went by, I realized that the team and coach were really into their Bible study and prayer and reciting Psalms before games. This is reflected positively in their character and conduct. The collective approach to spirituality brought positive energy that surprised me; but i know my jewish faith was and is the only true proven religion in the world.

I had some disagreements with the coach and G-d was sending me in a different direction. It seemed it was time to take a brief break from basketball, explore the world of philosophy and academics, and truly question what was out there ? and what I wanted out of life. I learned and researched more about Judaism and Israel. I enrolled in a study program abroad at Tel Aviv University, which changed my life. It was the first time I had been back in Israel since I was about 10 years old. I was energized by the people, the land, and their passion for life. After helping with the family clothing business, I knew my destiny was not to design or sell suits and ties. Instead, my soul was thirsty for the truth of life and missing the game I once loved. So, I decided to refocus on taking more credits and finishing up at the university.

It was a challenging journey, and I found that my soul was searching for more than just academics and basketball. I wanted the meaning of life. Nevertheless, I never gave up and worked hard at the game, and upon my graduation, I caught the eye of a sports agent. As a result, I was blessed with an opportunity to attend several professional camps and tryouts across America.

I was soon signed to play professional basketball in Israel. It was a wonderful time, but my passion waned after playing for several teams, plagued by injury, administrative wrangling, and political struggles and maneuvers within the basketball organizations. What was once true love is becoming all about the next paycheck. I realized playing professionally overseas meant I would have to consider playing in any part of the world, even in places where I would have to sacrifice my Jewish practices. I also discovered that leading an everyday family life and playing professional sports do not always match.

Then and there, I decided to take the plunge and sacrifice myself to the world of faith, God, and Judaism. I met some great educators and rabbis, finally beginning my journey to the Yeshiva world. I have learned a lot over these past years, and I am still learning. So, I decided to try to help inspire others from my experience and sought out coaching opportunities and my spiritual pursuits. I have fallen time and time again in my life, but each time I have used my faith to rise and become stronger than before. As King Solomon says in Proverbs

24:16, "The righteous person falls seven times and gets up. The evil person falls just once." Through challenges in our lives, GOD wants to purify us and make us even stronger!

I believe we are all great because GOD allows us to wake up each day and decide. We are all in this together, so make the adjustments, and let's get better. I'm currently helping people with their weight and wellness goals. I'm a certified trainer with the National Academy of Sports Medicine. I have trained alongside and worked with NBA, Euro, NCAA, and high school athletes. I used my personal and coaching experience to try to best help my clients. If you are interested in having help with your wellness goals, please email me at info@soulfit.com or see www.soulfit.com. I am humbled to share what I have learned with you. Thank you for your time.

GLOSSARY

1. **Emunah**—Deep faith and unwavering belief in God beyond logic.

2. **Bitachon**—Complete trust in God's plan and protection.

3. **Teshuvah** – Spiritual return or repentance; reconnecting with divine purpose.

4. **Neshama**—The divine soul or inner spiritual essence of a person.

5. **Yetzer Hara**—The negative inclination or selfish desire within human nature.

6. **Yetzer Hatov**—The good inclination that guides moral and spiritual behavior.

7. **Chesed**—Loving-kindness, compassion, or selfless giving.

8. **Shechinah**—The indwelling presence of God in the world.

9. **Ruach HaKodesh**—The Holy Spirit; divine inspiration or prophecy.

10. **Gan Eden**—The Garden of Eden; paradise or state of divine closeness.

11. **Gehinnom**—**Spiritual** purification realm; not eternal damnation but cleansing of the soul.

12. **Aliyah**—Ascending, both physically to Israel and spiritually to higher levels.

13. **Geulah**—Redemption; divine deliverance from exile and suffering.

14. **Mashiach**—The Messiah; the anointed one who brings ultimate redemption.

15. **Shamayim**—The heavens; the spiritual realm of divine reality.

16. **Tzedakah**—righteous giving; charity performed with justice and compassion.

17. **Halacha**—Jewish law; the collective body of spiritual and ethical commandments.

18. **Midrash**—**Rabbinic** commentary revealing deeper meanings in Scripture.

19. **Pardes**—Four levels of Torah interpretation: Peshat, Remez, Derash, and Sod.

20. **Sod**—The secret or mystical level of understanding in the Torah.

21. **Middot** – Character traits or ethical qualities cultivated for self-improvement.

22. **Ahavat Yisrael**—Love of one's fellow Jew; foundation of unity and kindness.

23. **Avodah**—Divine service; worship and spiritual work through daily acts.

24. **Simcha**—Joy or spiritual happiness that draws divine blessing.

25. **Shalom Bayit**—Peace in the home; harmony between family members.

26. **Olam HaBa**—"The World to Come"; the eternal spiritual existence after physical life.

27. **Mitzvot—Commandments** or divine instructions given in the Torah that guide moral, spiritual, and ethical behavior.

28. **Kedusha—holiness** or sanctification. *Kedusha* refers to the state of being **set apart for a sacred purpose**.

29. **Torah—Divine** teaching or law. The Torah is seen as **God's blueprint for living**, guiding moral conduct, faith, and the relationship between humanity and the Divine.

30. **Shema—The** *Shema* is the central declaration of Jewish faith; it affirms the oneness of God and the commitment to love and serve Him with all one's heart, soul, and might.

19. Partha—Fountched of human imagination. People, Armies, Desert and nations.

20. Sati—The depiction of the... comprehension of the world.

21. Noble—had a marriage in prith onal qualities supposed to be distinctive of all.

22. Above Divisions of everyone's relationship foundation of all individual thoughts.

23. ... —Divine service, worship and community work through ...

24. Anantha—Joy, spiritual happiness, pleasure, divine ...

25. Santanathya—Peace in the ... pity, harmony between human...

26. Ghar Hara—The Twofold Cosmic... The eternal spiritual brotherhood of physical life.

27. ... —Commandments of living, right moral growth in the total, the guide moral, spiritual, and ethical Sea of life.

28. Kedavsha—both as a justification As the system of the establishing set aside for a sacred purpose.

29. Torah—Divine teaching to live. The Torah is seen as God's blueprint for living guiding moral, spiritual, faith, and the relationship between humanity and the Divine.

30. Shema—The Shema is the central declaration of Jewish faith. It affirms the oneness of God and the commitment to love and serve God with all one's heart, soul, and might.

www.ingramcontent.com/pod-product-compliance
Lightning Source LLC
Chambersburg PA
CBHW052126270326
41930CB00012B/2782